◆ 药学实验系列教材 ◆

药物分析实验指导

（中英双语）

Experiment and Guidance for Pharmaceutical Analysis

徐新军 主编

中山大学出版社
SUN YAT-SEN UNIVERSITY PRESS

·广州·

图书在版编目（CIP）数据

药物分析实验指导：汉、英/徐新军主编．—广州：中山大学出版社，2022.3
（药学实验系列教材）
ISBN 978 - 7 - 306 - 07408 - 9

Ⅰ.①药…　Ⅱ.①徐…　Ⅲ.①药物分析—实验—汉、英　Ⅳ.①R917 - 33

中国版本图书馆 CIP 数据核字（2022）第 024862 号

YAOWU FENXI SHIYAN ZHIDAO

出　版　人：王天琪
策划编辑：陈　慧　鲁佳慧
责任编辑：鲁佳慧
封面设计：曾　婷
责任校对：吴茜雅
责任技编：靳晓虹
出版发行：中山大学出版社
电　　话：编辑部 020 - 84110283，84113349，84111997，84110779，84110776
　　　　　发行部 020 - 84111998，84111981，84111160
地　　址：广州市新港西路 135 号
邮　　编：510275　　传　　真：020 - 84036565
网　　址：http：//www. zsup. com. cn　E-mail：zdcbs@ mail. sysu. edu. cn
印　刷　者：广州市友盛彩印有限公司
规　　格：787mm×1092mm　1/16　13.25 印张　320 千字
版次印次：2022 年 3 月第 1 版　2022 年 3 月第 1 次印刷
定　　价：49.80 元

如发现本书因印装质量影响阅读，请与出版社发行部联系调换

本书编委会

主　　编　徐新军

编写人员　徐新军　姚美村　刘　丹　陶俊妃　陈缵光

前　言

　　药物分析是药学专业的一门专业课程，药物分析实验是该课程的重要组成部分，约占整个教学时数的一半。根据教学大纲，药物分析实验课程要求学生能够较系统地掌握《中国药典》常用的分析方法和实验技术，包括药物鉴别、杂质检查、含量测定等基本原理和常用仪器的操作技术，从而培养学生独立进行药品检验及质量标准制订工作的能力。

　　本书的编写主要依据《中国药典》所收载的内容，从中选出具有代表性的一些药品及方法。本书中的实验，从分析对象看，包括化学药物、中药制剂、体内生物样品；从实验方法看，包括容量分析法、电位滴定法、紫外分光光度法、高效液相色谱法、气相色谱法等，同时也将新技术的应用——微流控芯片分析法引入实验，让学生既掌握常规的药品检测方法，又了解学科发展的前沿，提高学习的兴趣；从实验内容看，包括药品质量控制与体内药物分析方法的建立；从剂型看，包括原料药、片剂、针剂及胶囊等。

　　本课程的教学，既能增强学生对药物分析理论知识的理解，又能规范其基本操作；在设计性实验环节培养学生进行药物分析研究的基本思路和独立从事药物分析研究的基本实验技能。

　　为了达到教学大纲的要求，学生课前必须认真预习，明确实验目的，了解实验内容与方法，并结合课堂教学掌握实验的基本原理；实验中要有严谨的科学态度和实事求是的作风，严格操作，正确使用仪器，认真观察实验现象，详细做好原始记录。实验数据不得任意涂改，实验报告要求书写正确整洁；严格遵守实验室规章制度，注意安全，保持室内卫生。

　　为方便学生在实验课学习过程中熟悉《中国药典》的内容及常用药物的分析知识，本书第二章摘录了常用的《中国药典》知识，附录二选录了《中国药典》与《美国药典》收载的一相同的个论，以供学生了解药典的内容编排，便于比较学习，培养其熟练使用《中国药典》并严格按照《中国药典》的规定进行操作的良好习惯。

　　本书的编写得到中山大学设备处实验教学研究（改革）基金的支持，特此致谢。

　　因编者时间有限，书中难免有疏漏错误之处，敬请读者批评指正。

编　者

2021 年 3 月

目　录

上　编　药物分析实验的基本知识

第一章　药物分析实验的基本要求

Chapter 1　Basic Requirements for Pharmaceutical Analysis Experiments ············ 3

第一节　实验须知 ················ 3

Section 1　Experimental Notes ················ 4

第二节　实验受伤应急处理 ················ 6

Section 2　Emergency Treatments of Experimental Injuries ················ 7

第三节　药物分析实验课程教学大纲 ················ 8

Section 3　Syllabus of Pharmaceutical Analysis Experiments Course ········ 10

第四节　实验数据的记录、处理和实验报告 ········ 14

Section 4　Recording, Processing of Experimental Data and Experimental Report ················ 15

第二章　药物分析实验常用仪器及方法简介

Chapter 2　Introduction of Commonly Used Instruments and Methods for Pharmaceutical Analysis Experiments ················ 17

第一节　常用玻璃仪器的洗涤和干燥 ················ 17

Section 1　Washing and Drying for Common Glassware ················ 19

第二节　电子天平的使用和维护 ················ 21

Section 2　Use and Maintenance of Electronic Balance ················ 25

第三节　紫外 – 可见分光光度法 ················ 30

Section 3　Ultraviolet Visible Spectrophotometry ················ 33

第四节　薄层色谱法 ················ 36

Section 4　Thin Layer Chromatography（TLC） ·················· 40

第五节　高效液相色谱法 ··· 45

Section 5　High Performance Liquid Chromatography（HPLC） ············ 52

下　编　药物分析实验

实验一　容量仪器的校正 ·· 67

Experiment 1　The Calibration of Volumetric Instruments ··········· 71

实验二　葡萄糖的分析 ·· 75

Experiment 2　The Analysis of the Glucose ························ 81

实验三　苯甲酸钠的分析 ·· 90

Experiment 3　The Analysis of Sodium Benzoate ·················· 92

实验四　药物中特殊杂质的检查 ·· 95

Experiment 4　The Tests of Specified Impurities in Drugs ············ 100

实验五　复方丹参滴丸中冰片、丹参的薄层色谱法分析 ···················· 105

Experiment 5　TLC Analysis of Borneol and Salvia Miltiorrhiza in Compound
　　　　　　　Danshen Dripping Pills ···························· 108

实验六　甘油磷酸钠含量测定 ··· 112

Experiment 6　Assay of Sodium Glycerophosphate ················ 117

实验七　高效液相色谱法测定头孢氨苄胶囊含量 ························· 123

Experiment 7　Assay of Cephalexin Capsules by HPLC ············ 127

实验八　气相色谱法测定维生素 E 软胶囊含量 ······················· 132

Experiment 8　The Determination of Vitamin E Soft Capsules by Gas
　　　　　　　Chromatography ································ 135

实验九　微流控芯片分析法测定赖氨酸颗粒剂中赖氨酸的含量 ············· 139

Experiment 9　Determination of Lysine in Lysine Granules by Microfluidic Chip
　　　　　　　Analysis ·· 143

实验十　高效毛细管电泳分离检测苯磺酸氨氯地平对映异构体·················· 147

Experiment 10　High Performance Capillary Electrophoresis for Detection of
Amlodipine Besylate Enantiomers ······························· 150

实验十一　咖啡酸片尿药浓度的测定 ···································· 153

Experiment 11　Determination of Caffeic Acid Concentration in Urine ············ 156

实验十二　兔血浆中茶碱血药浓度的高效液相色谱法分析 ··············· 160

Experiment 12　Determination of Theophylline in Rabbit's Plasma by HPLC ······ 164

实验十三　设计性实验——对乙酰氨基酚片的含量测定 ················· 169

Experiment 13　Design Experiment—Determination of Acetaminophen Tablets
·· 171

附　录

附录一　《中国药典》（2020 年版）通则 9101 分析方法验证指导原则·············· 175

Appendix Ⅰ　*Chinese Parmacopoeia* 9101 Guidelines for Validation of Analytical
Method Adopted in Pharmaceutical Quality Specification ······ 182

附录二　《中国药典》《美国药典》质量标准选读（以对乙酰氨基酚原料为例）

Appendix Ⅱ　Selecting Monograph from ChP and USP（Take Paracetamol as
an Example） ··· 191

附录三　药物分析常用英语词汇

Appendix Ⅲ　Vocabulary Commonly Used in Pharmaceutical Analysis ············ 196

参考文献··· 200

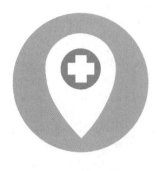

上编 | 药物分析实验的基本知识

第一章 药物分析实验的基本要求
Chapter 1 Basic Requirements for Pharmaceutical Analysis Experiments

第一节 实 验 须 知

实验是药物分析课程教学的重要组成部分，按教学大纲规定，实验课教学应做到：

（1）认真验证实验教材指定的药物分析理论，加深对本学科专业知识的理解。

（2）正确掌握实验教材中各类代表性药物的分析方法，熟练各种分析方法的操作技术，培养独立开展药物分析工作的能力。

（3）全面了解药物分析工作的性质和内容，培养严肃认真、实事求是的科学态度和工作作风。为提高实验课教学质量，参加实验课学习者应努力做到：

1）做好预习，明确每次实验的目的要求，弄懂原理和操作要点，预先安排好实验进程，估计实验中可能发生的问题及处理办法。每次实验课均应有准备地接受教师的提问。

2）严格按实验规程操作，虚心接受教师的指导，认真掌握操作技术，细心观察实验现象。进行讲义指定内容以外的实验或重做实验需要经教师批准。

3）进入实验室要携带《药物分析实验指导》及实验报告本。实验进程中应尊重实验事实，及时做好完整而确切的原始记录。要用钢笔或签字笔书写，字体端正。应直接将实验原始记录记在实验报告本上，绝不允许记于纸条上、手上或其他本子上再誊写，也不允许暂记在脑子里等下个数据一起记录。

原始记录是实验报告的一部分，尊重原始记录是必要的科学作风。记录本不得撕页，若记录有误，只能将写错处用双线划去（但要求仍能看清原来写错的数值），在其旁写上正确数据，不得涂改，涂改的原始记录无效。

4）防止试剂、药品污染，取用时应仔细观察标签和取用工具上的标志，杜绝错盖瓶盖或不随手加盖的现象发生。当不慎发生试剂污染时，应及时报告教师。公用试剂、药品应在指定位置取用。此外，取用后的试剂、药品不能再倒回原瓶。

5）爱护仪器，小心使用，破损仪器应及时登记报损、补发。动用精密仪器，需要经教师同意，用毕登记签名。

6）清楚各种安全设备（淋浴水龙头、洗眼喷淋、灭火器等）的放置位置及使用方法。

7）实验进行时，不得随便离开岗位，要密切注意实验的进展情况。进行可能发生危险的实验时，要根据实验情况采取必要的安全措施，如戴防护眼镜、面罩或橡胶手套等；使用易燃易爆化学试剂时，应远离火源，戴防护眼镜、防护手套等。进行实验时确保安全，时刻注意防火、防爆。发现事故苗头及时报告，不懂时不要擅自动手处理。

8）洗液一般只限于洗涤滴定管、吸量管、容量瓶等。使用时，应先用水冲洗仪器，沥至无滴水后，用洗液浸洗；其他玻璃仪器一般用肥皂或去污粉刷洗。注意节约使用蒸馏水，清洗玻璃仪器应遵守少量多次的原则。

9）做实验时应打开门窗和或换气设备，保持室内空气流通；加热易挥发有害液体，易产生严重异味、易污染环境的实验应在通风橱内进行。

10）各种气体钢瓶、煤气用毕或临时中断，都应立即关闭阀门，若发现漏气或气阀失灵，应停止实验，立即检查并修复，待实验室通风一段时间后，再恢复实验。禁止实验室内存在火种。需要循环冷却水的实验，应随时监测实验过程，不得随意离开，以免因减压或停水发生爆炸或着火事故。

11）使用电器时，谨防触电。不要在通电时用湿手或物接触电器或插头。实验完毕，应将电器的电源切断。

12）爱护公物，节约水、电、药品和试剂。将可回收利用的废溶剂回收至指定的容器中，不可任意弃去。实验所产生的化学废液应按有机、无机和剧毒等分类收集存放，严禁倒入下水道及水槽。

13）实验完毕应认真清理实验台，仪器洗净后放回原处，擦净台面，晾好抹布、毛刷，摆好凳子、锁好柜子，经教师同意后方可离开。值日生还应负责整理公用试剂台、打扫地面卫生、清除垃圾及废液缸中污物，并检查水、电、门、窗等安全事项。

14）认真总结实验结果，按指定格式完成实验报告，并按规定时间递交。

Section 1   Experimental Notes

Experiment is an important part of the teaching of pharmaceutical analysis course. According to the syllabus, the teaching of experiment course should be as follows:

(1) Carefully verify the theory of pharmaceutical analysis specified in the experimental textbook and deepen your understanding of professional knowledge of the subject.

(2) Correctly grasp the analysis methods of various representative drugs in the experimental textbook, be proficient in the operation techniques of various analysis methods, and cultivate the ability to carry out the pharmaceutical analysis work independently.

(3) Comprehensively understand the character and content of pharmaceutical analysis, and cultivate a serious, practical and realistic scientific attitude and work style. In order to improve the teaching quality of experiment course, learners participating in experiment course should strive to do as follows:

1) Before the experiment, students are required to prepare well, understand the principle and steps of the experiment, arrange the experimental process in advance, estimate the possible problems and solutions in the experiments. Every students should prepare to answer questions from teachers.

2) Strictly operate in accordance with the experimental procedures, accept the teacher's guidance modestly, master the operation techniques carefully, and observe the experimental phenomena carefully. Any experiments beyond the content specified in the handout or redo experiments should be approved by the teacher.

3) Enter the laboratory carrying the record book and *The Pharmaceutical Analysis Experimental Handout*. The experimental facts should be respected during the experiment, and complete and accurate original records should be made in time. Write with a pen, or a sign pen and keep the font correct. The original record of the experiment should be recorded directly in the experiment report, it is strictly prohibited to write it down on notes, hands or other books, then transcribe it or temporarily keep it in your mind to wait for the next data to be recorded together.

The original record is the part of the experiment report, and respect for the original record is a necessary scientific style. The record book is not allowed to tear pages. If the record is wrong, you can only cross the wrong line with a double line(but the original wrong words is still seen clearly), and write the correct data next to it. Don't alter it, the original altered record is invalid.

4) To prevent contamination of reagents and drugs, observe the labels and the marks on the tools carefully when taking them to prevent the wrong capping or not capping. Teachers should be promptly reported when reagent contamination occurs by accident. Public reagents and drugs should be taken at designated locations. In addition, the reagents and drugs taken can't be returned to the original bottle.

5) Take good care of the instruments and use them carefully. Damaged instruments should be registered for damage and reissued in time. The use of precision instruments requires the consent of the teacher and registered and signed after using.

6) Be sure to know where safe facilities(shower hydrant, eyewash and fire extinguisher etc.) are located.

7) Don't leave your post casually and pay close attention to the progress of the experiment, while the experiment is in progress. When conducting a potentially dangerous experiment, take necessary safety measures according to the experimental situation, such as wearing protective glasses, masks or rubber gloves. When using flammable and explosive chemical reagents, keep away from fire sources, wear protective glasses, protective gloves, etc. Ensure safety during the experiment and pay attention to fire prevention and explosion protection at all times. Report the accident signs in time, and don't handle them by yourself if

you don't know.

8) Chromic acid lotion is generally limited to washing burettes, pipettes, volumetric flasks, etc. When using it, the instrument should be washed with water first, and then soaked with washing liquid after no water dripping. Other glass instruments are generally washed with soap or detergent. Pay attention to saving distilled water, cleaning glass instruments should follow the principle of a small amount and multiple times.

9) When doing the experiment, doors, windows and/or ventilating equipments should be opened to maintain indoor air circulation. The experiments that heating volatile and harmful liquid, are liable to produce serious odor and pollute the environments should be conducted in a fume hood.

10) When all kinds of gas cylinders and gas are used up or temporarily interrupted, the valve should be closed immediately. If leakage or gas valve failure is found, the experiment should be stopped, checked and repaired immediately, and the experiment should be resumed after the laboratory is ventilated for a period of time. Tinder mustn't be in the laboratory. For experiments that require circulating cooling water, the progress of the experiment must be monitored at any time, and people mustn't leave casually to avoid decompression or stopping water to cause explosions and fire accidents.

11) When using electrical appliances, beware of electric shock. Don't touch electrical appliances or electrical pins with wet hands and objects while power is on. After the experiment is completed, the power of the appliance should be cut off.

12) Take care of public property and save water, electricity, drugs and reagents. Recyclable waste solvents are recycled into designated containers and can't be discarded arbitrarily. The chemical waste liquid produced in the experiment should be collected and stored according to the classification of organic, inorganic and highly toxic, and it is strictly prohibited to be poured into the sewer and the water tank.

13) Carefully clean the laboratory bench after the experiment. After the instrument is washed, put it back in place, wipe the table, dry the cloth and brush, place the stool and lock the cabinet, and leave with the teacher's consent. Students on duty should be responsible for arranging the public reagent table, cleaning the ground, removing garbage and waste from the waste liquid tank, and checking water, electricity, doors and windows and other safety matters before leaving.

14) Carefully summarize the experimental results, complete the experimental report according to the specified format, and submit it according to the prescribed time.

第二节　实验受伤应急处理

（1）强酸灼伤时，必须先用大量流水彻底冲洗，然后在皮肤上擦拭碱性药物。

（2）碱灼伤时，必须先用大量流水冲洗至皂样物质消失，然后用1%～2%醋酸或3%硼酸溶液进一步冲洗。

（3）酚灼伤皮肤，不可直接用水冲，以免加重创伤。可用浸了甘油或聚乙二醇与酒精的混合液（7∶3）的棉花除去污物后，再用清水冲洗干净，然后用饱和硫酸钠溶液湿敷。

（4）火/热水等引起的小面积烧伤、烫伤，必须用冷水冲洗30 min以上，然后用烧伤膏涂抹。

（5）火/热水等引起的大面积烧伤、烫伤，必须用湿毛巾、湿布、湿棉被覆盖，然后送医院进行处理。

（6）一般烫伤和烧伤，不要弄破水泡，在伤口处用95%的酒精轻涂伤口，涂上烫伤膏或涂一层凡士林油，再用纱布包扎。

（7）实验中遇到一般割伤，应立即清除伤口内异物，保持伤口干净，并用酒精棉清除伤口周围的污物，涂上外伤膏或消炎粉。

（8）实验中遇到严重割伤，可在伤口上部10 cm处用纱布扎紧，减缓血流，并立即送医院。

Section 2　Emergency Treatments of Experimental Injuries

（1）In the case of strong acid burns, rinse thoroughly with plenty of running water at first, and then wipe the alkaline medicine on the skin.

（2）In the case of alkali burns, rinse with a large amount of running water until the soap-like substance disappears at first, and then further rinse with 1% to 2% acetic acid or 3% boric acid solution.

（3）When the skin is burned by phenol, don't wash it directly with water to avoid further trauma. Use cotton soaked with glycerin or a mixture of polyethylene glycol and alcohol(7∶3) to remove the dirt, rinse it with water, and then wet with a saturated sodium sulfate solution.

（4）For small areas of burns and scalds caused by fire or hot water, rinse with cold water for more than 30 minutes, and then apply with the burn cream.

（5）For large areas of burns and scalds caused by fire or hot water, cover with wet towels, wet cloths, and wet quilts, and then send him to the hospital for treatment.

（6）For general scalds and burns, don't break the blisters. Lightly smear the wound with 95% ethanol, apply scalding cream or a layer of petroleum jelly, and wrap with gauze.

（7）In the case of general cuts during the experiment, immediately remove the foreign body in the wound, keep the wound clean, and use alcohol cotton to remove the dirt around the wound, and apply wound ointment or anti-inflammatory powder.

（8）In the case of severe cuts during the experiment, use gauze to tie tightly at the top 10 cm of the wound to slow down the bleeding and send to the hospital immediately.

第三节　药物分析实验课程教学大纲

课程名称（中文）：药物分析实验

课程名称（英文）：Pharmaceutical Analysis Experiments

开课时间：三年级下学期

适用专业：药学专业

先修课程：无机化学、有机化学、分析化学、生物化学

一、课程简介与基本要求

药物分析学是实践性很强的学科，药物分析实验是药物分析学的实验课程。它以典型药物的检验及常用的药物分析方法为主要内容，通过实验课的学习，学生应进一步树立药品质量的观念，掌握常用的药物鉴别、检查与含量测定方法的原理和实验操作技能，培养分析问题和解决问题的能力，培养严谨、认真的科学作风，为今后的工作打下良好的基础。

药物分析实验的任务是培养学生树立强烈的药品质量观念，熟悉药品检验工作的基本程序，掌握常用的药物分析方法。通过学习，学生应达到以下要求：

（1）全面了解药物分析工作的程序及要求。

（2）掌握药物分析常用方法的原理及操作技术。

（3）能运用本课程基本理论及有关专业知识分析和解决实验中的问题。

（4）培养实事求是的科学态度和严谨认真的工作作风。

二、课程实验目的与要求

药物分析实验课是培养学生掌握基本操作技能的重要教学环节。通过有限的教学时数，经精心安排的实验内容的训练，学生应了解药品质量控制的全貌和建立分析方法的一般思路。过硬的基本操作技能是进行药品质量控制与药品质量研究的基本条件，也是保证药品质量真正符合法定标准的必要条件。如果因操作技术问题，将合格产品检验成"不合格品"，势必给生产厂家造成不必要的损失；若将不合格产品检验成"合格产品"，则会使劣质药品进入流通领域，危害人民的健康。掌握基本技能的关键在于"三严"，即严肃的态度、严密的方法和严格的要求。学生应珍惜实验训练机会，在实验过程中勤动手、勤思考。本课程的教学方式是在教师的指导下，由学生自己动手完成有关的实验。为提高实验课教学效率，必须做到如下九点：

（1）课前做好预习。明确该次实验的目的要求，弄懂原理及操作要点，考虑实验中必须注意的事项、实验的顺序、所需的仪器及必要的准备。每次实验课应有准备地接受指导教师的提问。

（2）要准备一个实验记录本，在对药物进行分析时，应将全部数据准确及时地用钢笔或签字笔记录于记录本上，绝不允许记于小纸条上或实验讲义上，甚至手掌上。原始记录是实验报告的组成部分，尊重实验原始记录是必要的科学作风，绝不允许擅自涂改记录本内任何数据，如为笔误，仅能以钢笔或签字笔将写错处划去（但要求能看清原来数据），再重写一次。实验完毕，应书写实验报告，并根据检验结果做出明确的结论。

（3）在实验中要养成整洁、细致、准确的优良习惯，切实严格遵守操作规程，注意基本操作与对实验现象的观察分析。

（4）随时都要有量的概念。任何一项含量测定均要同时做两份，两次测定结果应相符。绝不允许伪造或估计一个数据，两次结果不能做依据时，应重新测定一次。

（5）实验课不得随便旷课，或相互调课。实验期间不得擅自离开实验室，有急事须经指导教师同意后方可离开。实验报告必须按规定时间上交给教师以进行批改。

（6）实验时应避免试剂污染、试剂瓶盖错盖或不随手加盖的现象发生。当不慎发生试剂污染时，应以负责的态度及时处理。

（7）爱护公物，移物归位，节约水电，公用药品、试剂、仪器等用后应及时归位，仪器用后应洗净，破损仪器要及时登记。

（8）实验期间确保安全，应经常注意防火、防爆。

（9）实验完毕，做好各自实验台的清洁工作，值日生应做好实验室的卫生清洁工作及检查水、电、门、窗等安全事项。

三、主要仪器设备

分析天平（0.01 mg、0.1 mg、0.01 g）、烘箱、酸式滴定管、紫外分光光度计、气相色谱仪、比色管、检砷瓶、旋光仪、折光仪、pH/mV 计、原子吸收分光光度计、高效液相色谱仪、毛细管电泳仪、微流控芯片、马弗炉、真空干燥箱。

四、实验方式与基本要求

要求如实做好实验记录，不弄虚作假，正确处理实验数据，并做出结论。实验报告应格式规范，书写工整，表述科学、简洁。

五、考核与报告

根据学生的预习、实验操作、实验结果、报告书写及科学作风等方面的情况评定成绩。

平时实验占 70%，考查性实验占 30%。

六、说明

（1）药物分析实验是一门对实验技术有较高要求的课程。对于痕量和超痕量物质的分析，要获得正确可靠的结果，必须进行严格、规范的训练，并养成良好的科研工作作风。因此，对课程中的技能技术性内容，除单独进行必要的药品检验标准操作规范（SOP）训练外，还要将其融入综合与设计实验中，通过反复强化练习，达到牢固掌握"量"的概念和超痕量分析实验技能的目的。

（2）在课程的教学过程中，将不断深化和扩展教学内容。结合药学学科、《中国药典》的发展趋势与本院教师的最新科研成果，对实验课程内容进行更新，从而使课程的发展紧跟学科的发展，使学生及时接触学科前沿。

（3）结合实验教学进度，安排相应的开放实验。开放实验以科学研究实验为主，其内容可以由教师提供，或学生自带课题。通过实验室的全面开放，一方面可以加强学生创新意识与创新能力的培养，有利于优秀学生的成长与个性发展；另一方面可以使实验动手能力较差的学生得到更多的锻炼机会，从而提高其实验技能。

（4）科学研究型实验主要为药学专业优秀学生开设。其目的是让学生通过完成这类实验，对科学研究的方法有一个较为全面的认识，同时也激发学生热爱科学、追求真理的热情；另外，研究型实验可真正使学生尽早接触科学研究工作，使其创新意识、创新精神和创新能力在实践中得到培养与提高。

Section 3　Syllabus of Pharmaceutical Analysis Experiments Course

Course name(Chinese)：药物分析实验

Course name(English)：Pharmaceutical Analysis Experiments

Start time: the next semester of third grade

Applicable specialty: Pharmaceutical Science

Prerequisite courses: Inorganic Chemistry, Organic Chemistry, Analytical Chemistry, Biochemistry

1　Course Introduction and Basic Requirements

Pharmaceutical analysis is a highly practical subject, and pharmaceutical analysis experiments is an experiment course in pharmaceutical analysis. It focuses on the test of typical drugs and frequently-used methods of pharmaceutical analysis. Through the study of experiment course, students can further establish the concept of drug quality, master the principles and experimental operation skills of frequently-used identification, tests, and determination of drugs, cultivate the ability to analyze and solve problems, rigorous and serious scientific style, and lay a good foundation for the future.

The task of pharmaceutical analysis experiments is to train students to establish a strong concept of drug quality, to be familiar with the basic procedures of drug testing, and to master common methods of drug analysis. Students should meet the following requirements after the study:

(1) Understand the procedures and requirements for pharmaceutical analysis comprehensive.

(2) Master the principles and operating techniques of frequently-used methods for pharmaceutical analysis.

(3) Be able to use the basic theory and related professional knowledge of this course to analyze and solve problems in the experiments.

(4) Cultivate the practical and realistic scientific attitude, the rigorous and serious work style.

2　Experimental Purpose and Requirements of Course

The pharmaceutical analysis experiments course is an important teaching link to train students to master basic operation skills. Through limited teaching hours and carefully arranged training of experimental contents, students can understand the complete picture of drug quality control and general ideas for establishing analytical methods. Excellent basic operation skills are the basic conditions for drug quality control and drug quality research and the necessary conditions to ensure that the drug quality truly meets legal standards. If a qualified product is inspected as a "non-conforming product" due to operational technical problems, it will inevitably cause unnecessary losses to the manufacturers; if a non-conforming product is inspected as a "qualified product", it will make the inferior drugs enter the circulation field and harm the people's health. The key to master basic skills is the "three strictness", that is, the serious attitude, strict methods and strict requirements. Students are required to cherish the opportunity for experimental training, practice and think frequently during the experiment. The teaching method of this course is under the guidance of the teacher, and the students complete the relevant experiments by themselves. In order to improve the teaching efficiency of experiment courses, the following points must be done:

(1) Do a preview before class. Clarify the purpose and requirements of the experiment, understand the principles and operation points, consider the items that must be paid attention to in the experiment, the sequence of the experiment, the required equipments and the necessary preparations. Students should prepare to answer questions from the teacher in each experimental class.

(2) Prepare an lab notebook. When analyzing the drug, all the data should be accurately and timely recorded on the record book with a pen, never allow it to be written on a small note or experimental handout or even on the palm. The original record is an integral part of the experiment report, respecting the original record of the experiment is a necessary scientific

style. It is forbidden to alter any data in the record without authorization. If it is a typo, you can only erase the mistake with a pen(but the original data must be seen clearly), and rewrite it again. After the experiment is completed, an experimental report should be written and a clear conclusion should be drawn based on the test results.

(3) Develop a neat, meticulous, and accurate habit in the experiment. Strictly abide by the operating regulations and pay attention to the observation and analysis of basic operations and experimental phenomena.

(4) Always have the concept of quantity. Any determination of content must be done in two copies at the same time, the results of the two determinations should be consistent. It is never allowed to forge or estimate a piece of data. If the two results can't be used as the basis, it should be measured again.

(5) Don't be absent from class or transferred to each other in experiment class. During the experimental period, it is forbidden to leave the laboratory without permission. If someone have to leave in case of emergency, he should get permission of the teacher. The experimental report must be submitted to the teacher for correction at the prescribed time.

(6) Avoid the phenomenon of contamination of reagents, wrong cap of reagent bottle cap or no cap during the experiment. When reagent contamination occurs accidentally, it should be handled in time with a responsible attitude.

(7) Care for public things, move things in place and save water and electricity. Public medicine reagents or instruments should be returned in time after use, the instruments should be washed after use, and damaged instruments should be registered in time.

(8) Be sure of safety during the experiment, always pay attention to the prevention of fire and explosion.

(9) After the experiment is completed, do the cleaning of the respective laboratory table. The students on duty should do the sanitary cleaning of the laboratory and check the water, electricity, doors, windows and other safety matters.

3　Main Instruments

Analytical balance(0. 01 mg, 0. 1 mg, 0. 01 g) , oven, acid buret, UV spectrophotometer, gas chromatograph, colorimetric tube, arsenic detector, polarimeter, refractometer, pH/mV meter, atomic absorption spectrophotometer, high performance liquid chromatography, capillary electrophoresis, microfluidic chip, muffle furnace, vacuum drying oven.

4　Experimental Procedures and Basic Requirements

It is required to make good experimental records without fraud, correctly handle experimental data and draw conclusions. The experimental report should be standard in format, neat in writing and scientific and concise in expression.

5 Assessment and Report

The students' marks are judged according to their preview, experimental operation, experimental results, reports written and scientific style, etc.

The normal experiment accounts for 70% and the experiment examination accounts for 30%.

6 Explanation

(1) "Pharmaceutical Analysis Experiments" is a course with higher requirements on experimental technology. For the analysis of trace and ultra-trace materials, to obtain correct and reliable results, strict standard training and a good scientific research work style must be carried out. Therefore, in addition to the necessary standard training on the standard operation procedure(SOP) for drug quality control, the technical content of the course is also integrated into the synthesis and design experiments. Through repeated practice, the purpose of firmly grasping the concept of "quantity" and the experimental skills of ultra-trace analysis are achieved.

(2) The teaching content will be continuously deepened and expanded during the course of teaching. Combining the development trend of the pharmacy discipline and ChP with the latest scientific research results of the teachers of the college, the content of the experiment course is updated, so that the development of the course closely follows the development of the discipline and students can contact the frontier of the discipline in a timely manner.

(3) According to the experimental teaching progress, arrange corresponding open experiments. Open experiments are mainly based on scientific research experiments. The content can be provided by teachers or students who can bring their own topics. Through the comprehensive opening of the laboratory. On the one hand, it can strengthen the cultivation of students' innovative consciousness and innovation ability, which is conducive to the growth and personality development of outstanding students. On the other hand, it can allow students with poor experimental skills to get more exercise opportunities, thereby improve their experimental skills.

(4) Scientific research experiments are mainly set up for excellent students majoring in pharmacy. The purpose is to enable students to have a comprehensive understanding of scientific research methods by completing such experiments, and also to stimulate students' passion on science and the pursuit of truth. In addition, research-based experiments really enable students to get in touch with scientific research as soon as possible, so that their innovative consciousness, spirit and ability can be cultivated and improved in practice.

第四节　实验数据的记录、处理和实验报告

一、实验数据的记录

学生应有专门的实验记录本并标上连续页码，不能随便撕去任何一页，绝不允许将实验数据记录在小纸片上或随意记在任何其他地方。

实验过程中所得的各种测量数据及现象，应及时、准确而清楚地记录下来。记录实验数据时，要有严谨的科学态度，实事求是，切忌夹杂主观因素，绝不能随意拼凑和伪造数据；若发现数据读错、算错而需要改动时，可将该数据用两横线划去，另起一行写上准确的数据。

记录实验数据时，保留有效数字的位数应和所用仪器的准确程度相适应，若用万分之一分析天平称量时，应记录至 0.000 1 g，滴定管和移液管的读数应记录至 0.01 mL。

实验记录上的每一个数据都是测量结果，因此重复观测时，即使数据完全相同也应记录下来。

二、分析数据的处理

实验中测得的一组数据，对其中的可疑数据是保留还是舍弃，可用 Q 检验法或 Grubbs 法进行检验并决定取舍，然后计算出其平均值，同时还应把分析结果的精密度表示出来。分析结果的精密度可用相对平均偏差、标准偏差（SD）及相对标准偏差（RSD）表示。

三、实验报告

实验报告一般包括下列内容：

（1）实验名称、实验日期、同组人员名字、温度、湿度。

（2）目的要求。

（3）方法原理：简要地用文字和化学反应式说明。

（4）操作步骤：可简明扼要写出，或用流线图表示。

（5）实验数据及处理：应用文字、表格、图形将数据表示出来，并根据实验要求按相应公式计算出分析结果和分析结果的精密度。

（6）问题及讨论：对实验中观察到的现象及实验结果进行分析和讨论。若实验失败，应寻找失败的原因，总结经验教训，必要时补做，以提高分析问题和解决问题的能力。

Section 4　Recording, Processing of Experimental Data and Experimental Report

1　Recording of Experimental Data

Students should have special lab notebooks, which mark the page number. They can't tear off any page, it is prohibited to record the experiment data on a small piece of paper or record it anywhere.

The various measurement data and phenomena obtained during the experiment should be timely recorded accurately and clearly. When recording the experimental data, you must have a rigorous scientific attitude, be practical and realistic, and avoid mixing with subjective factors. We should never randomly assemble and falsify the data. If you find that the data is wrongly read or miscalculated and you need to change it, you can use two horizontal lines to cross out the data and write the accurate data on another line.

When recording the experimental data, the number of significant digits retained should be compatible with the accuracy of the instrument used. For example, when weighing with a ten-thousandth analytical balance, it should be recorded to 0.000 1 g, and the readings of the burette and pipette should be recorded to 0.01 mL.

Every data recorded on the lab notebook is the result of measurement, so when repeated observation, even if the data is identical, it should be recorded.

2　Processing of Analytical Data

For a group of data measured in the experiment, whether to keep or discard the suspicious data, it can be determined by the Q-test or Grubbs method, and then the average value can be calculated. At the same time, the precision of the analysis results should be expressed. The precision of the analysis results can be expressed by relative average deviation, standard deviation(SD) and relative standard deviation(RSD).

3　Experiment Reports

Experiment reports generally include the following:

(1) Experiment topic, experiment date, name of the students in the same group, temperature, humidity.

(2) Purposes and requirements.

(3) Methods and principles: it is briefly described in words and chemical reaction formula.

(4) Operation procedures: it can be written concisely, or represented by a flow chart.

(5) Experimental data and processing: the data can be represented by words, tables or figures, and the analysis results and the precision of the analysis results are calculated

according to the experimental requirements and corresponding formulas.

(6) Questions and discussions: the phenomena and experimental results observed in the experiment are analyzed and discussed. If the experiment fails, you should find the cause of the failure, summarize the experience and lessons, and make up experiment if necessary, so as to improve the ability to analyze and solve problems.

第二章 药物分析实验常用仪器及方法简介
Chapter 2 Introduction of Commonly Used Instruments and Methods for Pharmaceutical Analysis Experiments

第一节 常用玻璃仪器的洗涤和干燥

一、仪器的洗涤

在药物分析工作中，洗涤玻璃仪器不仅是一项实验前的预备工作，也是一项技术性的工作。仪器洗涤是否符合要求，对分析结果的准确度和精密度均有影响。洗涤仪器的方法很多，应当根据实验的要求、污物的性质和玷污的程度来选择。一般有下列几种洗涤方法。

（一）用水刷洗

此法既可洗去溶于水的物质，又可使附着在仪器上的尘土和不溶性物质脱落下来，但对油污洗涤效果并不好。洗刷时，应选用合适的刷子，如用试管刷去洗烧杯，就不合适，因为试管刷太细，不易将烧杯底洗净。若刷子顶端无毛，则不宜使用，易损坏玻璃器皿。

（二）用去污粉或合成洗涤剂刷洗

市售的餐具洗洁精是以非离子表面活性剂为主要成分的中性洗液，可配制成 $1\%\sim2\%$ 的水溶液，也可用 5% 的洗衣粉水溶液刷洗仪器，它们都有较强的去污能力，必要时可用温热的洗涤剂或短时间浸泡。经洗涤后的仪器倒置时，水流出后的器壁应不挂水珠，之后再用少许纯水冲洗仪器 3 次，洗去自来水带来的杂质。

（三）浓硫酸－重铬酸钾洗涤液（又称铬酸洗液）

这种洗液具有很强的氧化性，对有机物和油污的去污能力特别强，适用于一些对洁净程度要求较高的定量器皿（如滴定管、容量瓶、移液管等）及一些形状特殊、不能用刷子刷洗的仪器。

它的具体配制方法：称取 10 g 研细的重铬酸钾固体，加热溶于 20 mL 水中，待冷却后，边搅拌边缓慢地加入 180 mL 浓 H_2SO_4（切勿将溶液加入浓 H_2SO_4！），冷却后移入具塞瓶中保存。使用洗液的方法及注意事项如下：

（1）使用洗液前，应先用水刷去外层污物，并用水冲洗内层污物。冲洗完毕后应尽量将仪器内的残存水倒掉，避免水把洗液稀释，降低其氧化能力。

（2）用洗液时，首先倒入仪器 $1/5\sim1/4$ 体积的洗液，然后慢慢地将仪器倾斜旋转，使仪器的内壁全部为洗液润湿，反复操作 1～2 次；再将洗液倒回贮存瓶中，将仪器倒置一会儿，让残存的洗液流尽，后用水将附着在内壁的洗液冲洗干净；最后用少量蒸馏水或去离子水洗去残存在自来水中的 Ca^{2+}、Mg^{2+}、Cl^- 等离子，反复此操作 3 次左右。若仪器较脏，可将洗液充满整个仪器，浸泡一段时间，或用热洗液洗，去污能力更强。

（3）洗液可重复使用，直至洗液变成绿色（$Cr_2O_7^{2-}$ 中的 Cr^{6+} 被还原成 Cr^{3+}），才失效报废。

（4）洗液变稀时，将会有重铬酸钾析出，氧化能力将有所降低，但仍可使用。也可将其蒸浓后再用。洗液具有很强的腐蚀性，会灼伤皮肤和破坏衣物。若不慎把洗液洒在衣物上，应立即用水冲洗；若洒在桌上，应立即用抹布揩去，抹布用水洗净。

（5）Cr（Ⅵ）有毒，清洗残留在仪器上的洗液时，第一、第二遍水不要倒入下水道，应倒入废液缸中统一处理，以免污染环境。

（四）氢氧化钠 - 高锰酸钾洗液

此洗液适用于洗油腻及有机物较多的仪器。配制方法：称取 4 g 高锰酸钾溶于少量水中，缓慢地加入 100 mL 10% NaOH 溶液即成。此洗液会腐蚀玻璃，不宜洗定量精密仪器，且洗后会有二氧化锰沉淀，其可用浓盐酸或亚硫酸钠溶液洗去。

上述几种洗涤方法，可根据不同的要求进行选择。洗净的仪器应不挂水珠，将仪器倒置时，水会顺着器壁流下，器壁上只留下一层既薄又均匀的水膜。注意，手上有汗或油脂，拿洗净的仪器应捏上口边缘，否则仪器外壁易挂水珠。外壁水珠用手或滤纸可抹去或移去，内壁水珠不可抹去或移去。

二、仪器的干燥

仪器的干燥一般有以下三种方法。

（一）烘干

将洗净的仪器倒置或平放于搪瓷盘中，放入电热干燥箱（即烘箱）中烘干。最好同时鼓风，使烘干速度加快。注意，准确定量的仪器如量瓶、移液管、滴定管等不宜烘干，应倒置，沥干水分。

（二）晾干

将洗净的仪器倒置或平放于干净的实验柜内（最好放在干净的搪瓷盘中再放入柜内）或仪器架上晾干。

（三）吹干

用吹风机将洗净的仪器吹干。有时为了加快吹干速度，先用少量酒精或丙酮与仪器内的水互溶，倒出，然后用冷风吹干。由于丙酮与酒精沸点较低，挥发快，易吹干。

Section 1 Washing and Drying for Common Glassware

1 Washing of Glass Instruments in Common Use

In the pharmaceutical analysis work, it is not only a preparatory work before the experiment to wash the glassware, but also a technical work. Whether the washing work meets the requirements has impacts on the degree of accuracy and precision of the analysis results. There are many washing methods, which should be selected according to the requirements of the experiment, the nature of the dirt and the pollution level. Generally there are the following washing methods:

1.1 Scrub with Water

This method can not only wash away water-soluble substances, but also allow dust and insoluble substances attached to the instrument to fall off. But it's unsuitable for the oil contamination. When washing, you must use a suitable brush. It is not appropriate for you to wash the beaker with a test tube brush for the reason that it is too thin to clean the bottom of the beaker. It should not be used if the tip of the brush is lint-free, as it can easily damage the glassware.

1.2 Scrub with Detergent or Synthetic Detergent

The commercially available dishwashing detergent is a neutral detergent with non-ionic surfactants as the main components. It can be formulated into a $1\% \sim 2\%$ aqueous solution. We can also scrub the instruments with a 5% washing powder aqueous solution. These solutions all have strong decontamination ability, and can be warmed or soaked for a short time if necessary. When the washed instrument is upside down, after the water flows out, the wall of the device should be free of water droplets. At this point, the instrument should be rinsed by three times with a little pure water to wash away the impurities brought by the tap water, and be ready to use.

1.3 Concentrated Sulfuric Acid-potassium Dichromate Scrubbing Solution (Chromic Acid Lotion)

This lotion has a strong oxidizing property, and it has a particularly strong decontamination ability to organic compounds and oil contamination. It is suitable for some quantitative vessels(such as burettes, volumetric flasks, pipettes, etc.) that require a high degree of cleanliness, as well as some instruments with special shapes that cannot be washed with a brush.

Its specific preparation method is as follows : Weigh 10 g of finely ground solid potassium dichromate, heat and dissolve in 20 mL of water. After cooling, slowly add 180 mL of concentrated sulfuric acid while stirring(do not add the solution to concentrated sulfuric acid).

After cooling, store the lotion in a bottle with stopper. The methods and precautions for using the lotion are as follows:

(1) Before using the lotion, first brush the outer dirt and flush the inner dirt with water. After flushing, the residual water in the instrument should be drained as far as possible to avoid diluting the lotion with water and reducing its oxidation capacity.

(2) When using the lotion, first pour the lotion into about 1/5 to 1/4 of the volume of the instrument, and then slowly tilt the instrument to make the inner wall of the instrument moisten with the lotion. Repeat the operation once or twice. Pour the lotion back into the storage bottle, invert it for a while, let the remaining lotion run out, then rinse the lotion attached to the inner wall with water. Finally, wash away the remaining Ca^{2+}, Mg^{2+}, Cl^- in tap water with a small amount of distilled water or deionized water. Repeat this operation about three times. If the instrument is particularly dirty, you can fill the entire instrument with the lotion, soak it for a while, or wash it with hot lotion, which has stronger decontamination ability.

(3) The lotion can be reused until the lotion turns green(Cr^{6+} is reduced to Cr^{3+}) before it is invalidated.

(4) When the lotion becomes thinner, potassium dichromate will be precipitated, and the oxidation ability will become lower, but it can still be used. It can also be used after distillation and concentration. The lotion is highly corrosive and can burn skin and damage clothing if the lotion is accidentally spilled on the clothes, it should be washed immediately with water. If it is spilled on the table, it should be wiped off immediately with a rag, and the rag should be washed with water.

(5) Cr(Ⅵ) is poisonous. When cleaning the lotion remaining on the instrument, do not pour the first and second times of water into the sewer. Instead, pour it into a waste liquid tank to dispose of it uniformly, so as not to pollute the environment.

1.4 Sodium Hydroxide-potassium Permanganate Lotion

This kind of lotion is suitable for washing instruments with oil contamination and organic compounds. Its specific preparation method is as follows: Weigh 4 g of potassium permanganate and dissolve it in a small amount of water, and slowly add 100 mL of 10% NaOH solution. This kind of lotion can corrode glass, and it is not suitable to wash quantitative precision instruments. After washing, manganese dioxide will precipitate, and it can be washed away with concentrated hydrochloric acid or sodium sulfite solution.

Several washing methods have been introduced above, which can be selected according to different requirements. The washed instrument should be free of water droplets. When the instrument is turned upside down, water will flow down the container wall, leaving only a thin and uniform water film on the container wall. Note that if there is sweat or grease on your hands, you should pinch the edge of the mouth of the washed instrument, otherwise water droplets will easily hang on the outer wall of the instrument. Water drops on the outer wall can be removed by filter paper, water drops on the inner wall cannot be wiped off or removed.

2　Drying for Glass Instruments in Common Use

There are several ways to dry the instruments:

2.1　Stoving

Put the cleaned instrument upside down or flat on an enamel plate, put it in an oven to dry. It is best to blow air at the same time to make the drying speed faster. Note that accurate quantitative instruments such as measuring flasks, pipettes, and burettes should not be dried in this way. They should be inverted and drained of water.

2.2　Drying in the Air

Put the cleaned instrument upside down or place it in a clean laboratory cabinet (preferably in a clean enamel plate and then put it in the cabinet) or dry it on the instrument rack.

2.3　Blow Drying

Dry the cleaned instrument with a hair dryer. Sometimes, in order to speed up the drying speed, first use a small amount of alcohol or acetone to dissolve with the water in the instrument, pour it out, and then dry it with cold air. Because acetone and alcohol have low boiling points, they evaporate quickly and are easy to be blown dry.

第二节　电子天平的使用和维护

电子天平根据电磁力平衡原理直接称量，不需要砝码。放上称量物后，其在几秒钟内即达到平衡，显示读数，称量速度快、精度高。电子天平的支承点用弹性簧片取代机械天平的玛瑙刀口，用差动变压器取代升降枢装置，用数字显示代替指针刻度式。因此，电子天平具有使用寿命长、性能稳定、操作简便和灵敏度高的特点。此外，电子天平还具有自动校正、自动去皮、超载指示、故障报警及质量电信号输出等功能，且可与打印机、计算机联用，进一步扩展其功能，如统计称量的最大值、最小值、平均值及标准偏差等。由于电子天平具有机械天平无法比拟的优点，尽管其价格较贵，但越来越广泛地被应用于各个领域并逐步取代机械天平。

一、电子天平及其分类

电子天平的特点是称量准确、可靠，显示快速、清晰，并且具有自动检测系统、简便的自动校准装置及超载保护等装置。按电子天平的精度，其可分为以下四类。

（一）超微量电子天平

超微量天平的最大称量为 $2 \sim 5$ g，其精度为 0.000 1 mg 或 0.001 mg，如 Sartoruis

的 ME5 型电子天平，最大称量为 5.1 g，精度为 0.001 mg；Mettler 的 XPR2/AC 型电子天平的最大称量为 2.1 g，精度为 1μg。

（二）微量天平

微量天平的最大称量一般为 3～50 g，其分度值小于（最大）称量的 10^{-5}，如 Mettler 的 AT21 型电子天平及 Sartoruis 的 S4 型电子天平均属于此类。

（三）半微量天平

半微量天平的称量一般在 20～100 g，其分度值小于（最大）称量的 10^{-5}，如 Mettler 的 AE50 型电子天平和 Sartoruis 的 M25D 型电子天平均属于此类。

（四）常量电子天平

常量电子天平的最大称量一般为 100～200 g，其分度值小于（最大）称量的 10^{-5}，如 Mettler 的 AE200 型电子天平和 Sartoruis 的 A120S、A200S 型电子天平均属于常量电子天平。

二、电子天平的选用

选择电子天平应从电子天平的绝对精度（分度值）方面考虑其是否符合称量的精度要求。使用前首先看量程，根据实际最大称量范围来选择，最好比实际最大称重稍大一些；其次看精度，称重是否对质量要求很高。若需要精密称定，称取质量应准确至所取重量的千分之一。若是对炽灼残渣、干燥失重的测定，需恒重（≤0.3 mg），应选择万分之一天平；若需要精密称定质量为 10～100 mg 的样品，应选择十万分之一天平。

三、电子天平的校准

电子天平在使用前一般都应进行校准。校准方法分为内校准和外校准两种。德国生产的 Sartoruis，瑞士生产的 METTLER TOLEDO，上海生产的"FA"等系列电子天平均有校准装置。使用前必须仔细阅读说明书，按说明书要求进行校准。

四、电子天平的使用方法

（1）水平调节。电子天平在称量过程中会因为摆放位置不平而产生测量误差，称量精度越高误差就越大，因此，大多数电子天平具有调整水平的功能。

电子天平后面有一个水平仪气泡，需要调水平泡位于液腔中央，否则称量不准确。调好之后，应尽量不要搬动，否则，水平泡可能发生偏移，需要重新调整。电子天平一般有两个调平底座，一般位于后面，也有位于前面的。旋转这两个调平底座，就可以调整天平水平。

（2）预热。接通电源，预热至规定时间（天平长时间断电后再使用时，至少预热 30 min）后，开启显示器进行操作。

（3）开启显示器。轻按"ON"键，显示器全亮，约 2 s 后，显示天平的型号，然后是称量模式 0.000 0 g，读数时应关上天平门。

（4）天平基本模式的选定。天平通常为"Normal"模式，并具有断电记忆功能。使用时若改成了其他模式，使用后一经按"OFF"键，天平即恢复"Normal"模式。称量单位的设置等可按说明书进行操作。

（5）校准。天平安装后，第一次使用前，应对天平进行校准。因存放时间较长、位置移动、环境变化或未获得精确测量，天平在使用前一般都应进行校准操作。天平可采用外校准（有的电子天平具有内校准功能），具体按说明书操作。

（6）称量。按"TAR"键，显示为"0"后，置称量物于秤盘上，待数字稳定即显示器左下角的"0"消失后，即可读出称量物的质量。

（7）去皮称量。按"TAR"键清零，置容器于秤盘上，天平显示容器质量，再按"TAR"键，显示"0"，即去除皮重。再置称量物于容器中，或将称量物（粉末状物或液体）逐步加入容器中直至达到所需质量，待显示器左下角"0"消失，这时显示的是称量物的净质量。将秤盘上的所有物品拿开后，天平显示负值，按"TAR"键，天平显示"0.000 0 g"。若称量过程中秤盘上的总质量超过最大载荷（METTLER TOLED ME104E 型电子天平为 120 g）时，天平仅显示上部线段，此时应立即减小载荷。

（8）称量结束。若较短时间内还使用天平，一般不必按"OFF"键关闭显示器。实验全部结束后，关闭显示器，切断电源；若短时间内（如 1 h 内）还使用天平，可不必切断电源，再次使用时可省去预热时间。若当天不再使用天平，应拔下电源插头。

五、称量方法

常用的称量方法有直接称量法、固定质量称量法和减重称量法。

（一）直接称量法

直接称量法是将称量物放在天平盘上直接称量物体的质量。例如，称量小烧杯的质量，容量器皿校正中称量某量瓶的质量，重量分析实验中称量某坩埚的质量等，都使用这种称量法。

（二）固定质量称量法

固定质量称量法又称增量法，用于称量某一固定质量的试剂（如基准物质）或试样。这种称量操作的速度较慢，适用于称量不易吸潮、在空气中能稳定存在的粉末状或小颗粒（最小颗粒应小于 0.1 mg，以便容易调节其质量）样品。

使用固定质量称量法时应注意：若不慎加入的试剂超过指定质量，用药匙取出多余试剂。重复上述操作，直至试剂质量符合指定要求为止。须注意取出的多余试剂应弃去，不要放回原试剂瓶中。操作时不能将试剂散落于天平盘等容器以外的地方。称好的试剂必须定量地由称量瓶等容器直接转入接受容器，即定量转移。固定质量称量法适用于称量在空气中性质稳定、不吸水、不与氧气或二氧化碳反应等的物质，可用称量瓶、小烧杯等容器称量。

（三）减重称量法

减重称量法又称减量法，用于称量一定质量范围的样品或试剂。在称量过程中样品易吸水、易氧化或易与二氧化碳反应时，可选择此法。由于称取试样的质量是由两次称量之差求得，故也称减量法。药物分析实验中常用减量法称重。其操作过程如下：

（1）从干燥器中用纸带夹住称量瓶后取出称量瓶（也可直接佩戴棉质、硅胶或橡胶手套进行操作），注意不要让手指直接触及称量瓶和瓶盖，用纸片夹住称量瓶盖柄，打开瓶盖，用药匙加入适量试样（一般为称 1 份试样量的整数倍），盖上瓶盖，称出称量瓶加试样后的准确质量。

（2）将称量瓶从天平上取出，在接收容器的上方倾斜瓶身，用称量瓶盖轻敲瓶口上部使试样慢慢落入容器中，瓶盖始终不要离开接收容器上方。当倾出的试样接近所需量（可从体积上估计或试重得知）时，一边继续用瓶盖轻敲瓶口，一边逐渐将瓶身竖直，使黏附在瓶口上的试样落回称量瓶，然后盖好瓶盖，准确称其质量。

（3）两次质量之差，即为试样的质量。按上述方法连续递减，可称量多份试样。有时很难一次得到合乎质量范围要求的试样，可重复上述称量操作 1～2 次。

六、电子天平的维护与保养

电子天平室应避免阳光直射，最好选择阴面房间或采用遮光办法；应远离震源，如公路、振动机等振动机械，无法避免时应采取防震措施；应远离热源和高强电磁场等环境；工作室内温度应恒定，以 20 ℃左右为佳；工作室内的相对湿度以 45%～75% 为佳；工作室内应保持清洁干净，避免气流的影响；工作室内应无腐蚀性气体的影响；在使用前调整水平仪气泡至中间位置；电子天平应按说明书的要求进行预热；称量易挥发和具有腐蚀性的物品时，要盛放在密闭的容器中，以免腐蚀和损坏电子天平；经常对电子天平进行自校或定期外校，保证其处于最佳状态；如果电子天平出现故障应及时检修，不可带"病"工作；操作电子天平时不可过载使用以免损坏天平。

七、天平使用注意事项

（1）开启天平前，检查天平称量盘上及周围有无散落物质，用专用的天平刷清扫称量盘及天平箱内部。将称量盘垂直提起，检查有无散落物质，用刷清理后，小心地将称量盘安置回原位。

（2）不要将待测化学物质直接接触天平托盘，使用容器（如称量瓶、烧杯、量瓶或称量纸等）称量，尽量选用较小的容器称量。

（3）将待称量样品置于称量盘中央。

（4）称量物体时，关上天平门，防止空气扰动干扰读数。

Section 2　Use and Maintenance of Electronic Balance

The electronic balance is directly weighed without weight according to the principle of electromagnetic force balance. After putting on the weighing object, it will reach equilibrium within a few seconds, display readings. It has fast weighing speed and high accuracy. The supporting points of electronic balance use elastic reeds to replace the agate blades of mechanical balance, differential elevators to replace the lifting device, and digital indicators to replace the pointer scale type. Therefore, the electronic balance has the characteristics of long service life, stable performance, easy operation and high sensitivity. In addition, the electronic balance also has functions such as automatic calibration, automatic tare, overload indication, fault alarm, and quality electrical signal output. It can also be used with printers and computers to further expand its functions, such as statistical weighing of the maximum, minimum, average and standard deviation. Because electronic balance has advantages that mechanical balance cannot match, although they are more expensive, they are also increasingly widely used in various fields and gradually replace mechanical balance.

1　Electronic Balance and Its Classification

The electronic balance is characterized by accurate and reliable weighing, fast and clear display, and an automatic detection system, simple automatic calibration device, and overload protection device. According to the precision of the electronic balance, it can be divided into the following categories:

1.1　Ultramicro-Electronic Balance

The maximum weighing of this kind of balance is $2 \sim 5$ g. Its precision is 0.000 1 mg or 0.001 mg. For example, the ME5 type of Sartoruis has a maximum weight of 5.1 g and a precision of 0.001 mg. The XPR2 / AC type of Mettler has a maximum weight of 2.1 g and a precision of 1 μg.

1.2　Microelectronic Balance

Microelectronic balance has a measurement maximum of $3 \sim 50$ g. Its division value is less than 10^{-5} of the (maximum) weighing. For example, the AT21 type of Mettler and the S4 type of Sartoruis.

1.3　Semimicro-Electronic Balance

Semimicro-electronic balance has a measurement maximum of $20 \sim 100$ g. Its division value is less than 10^{-5} of the (maximum) weighing. For example, the AE50 type of Mettler and the M25D type of Sartoruis.

1.4　Constant Electronic Balance

This kind of balance has a measurement maximum of $100 \sim 200$ g. Its division value is less than 10^{-5} of the (maximum) weighing. For example, the AE200 type of Mettler and the A120S and A200S types of Sartoruis.

2　Selection of Electronic Balance

When selecting the kind of electronic balance, the absolute accuracy(division value) of the electronic balance should be considered to meet the accuracy requirements of the weighing. Firstly, pay attention to the measuring range of the balance before use, and select it according to your actual maximum weighing range. It is best for the measuring range to be slightly larger than your actual maximum weighing. Secondly, note the precision and check whether the weighing requires high precision. For precise weighing, the weight should be accurate to $1/1\,000$ of the weight taken. For the determination of flaming residue and loss on drying, constant weight(0.3 mg or less) is required, and a electronic balance($0.000\,1$ g) should be selected. For samples weighing $10 \sim 100$ mg, an electronic balance(0.01 mg) should be selected.

3　Calibration of Electronic Balance

Electronic balances should generally be calibrated before use. There are two calibration methods: internal calibration and external calibration. A series of electronic balances such as Sartoruis made in Germany, METTLER TOLEDO made in Switzerland, and "FA" made in Shanghai have calibration devices. Be sure to read the instructions carefully before use, and calibrate according to the instructions.

4　Instructions of Electronic Balance

4.1　Horizontal Adjustment

Electronic balances have measurement errors due to uneven placement during weighing. The higher the weighing precision, the greater the error. For this reason, most electronic balances provide the ability to adjust the level. There is a level bubble behind the electronic balance, it should be adjusted to the level bubble in the center of the liquid cavity, otherwise the weighing is not accurate. After adjustment, try not to move it, otherwise the level bubble may shift and need to be adjusted again. Electronic balances generally have two leveling bases, which are generally located at the rear and also at the front. You can adjust the balance level by rotating these two leveling bases.

4.2　Preheating

Turn on the power and preheat for a specified time(when the balance is powered off for a long time before using it, it needs to preheat for at least 30 min), then turn on the display for operation.

4.3　Turn on the Display

Press the "ON" key lightly, the display will be fully on. After about 2 s, the balance model is displayed, then the weighing mode is displayed of 0.000 0 g. The balance door should be closed when reading.

4.4　Selection of Basic Mode of the Balance

The balance is usually in "Normal" mode and has a power-off memory function. If you change to other modes during use, once you press the "OFF" key after use, the balance will return to the normal mode. The setting of the weighing unit can be operated according to the instructions.

4.5　Calibration

After the balance has been installed, it should be calibrated before the first use. Balances should generally be calibrated before use due to long storage time, location shifts, environmental changes, or inaccurate measurements. The balance adopts external calibration(some electronic balances have internal calibration function), and the specific operation is according to the instructions.

4.6　Weighing

After pressing the "TAR" key, when the display is zero, place the weighing object on the weighing pan. After the number is stable, that is, the "0" mark in the lower left corner of the display disappears, the mass of the weighing object can be read.

4.7　Tare Weighing

Press the "TAR" key to clear, place the container on the weighing pan. After the balance displaying the container weight, press the "TAR" key to display "0", that is, to remove the tare weight. Then place the weighing object in the container, or gradually add the weighing object(powder or liquid) to the container until the required quality is reached. When the "0" in the lower left corner of the display disappears, the net weight of the weighing object is displayed. After removing all the items on the weighing pan, the balance displays a negative value. Press the "TAR" key, and the balance displays 0.000 0 g. If the total mass on the weighing pan exceeds the maximum load during weighing(120 g for METTLER TOLED ME104E electronic balance), the balance only displays the upper line segment, and the load should be reduced immediately.

4.8　Ending Weighing

If the balance is still used for a short period of time, you generally do not need to press the "OFF" key to turn off the display. After all the experiments are over, turn off the display and cut off the power. If you use the balance for a short time(for example, within 1 h), you do not need to cut off the power, which can save the preheating time. If the balance is not to be used that day, unplug the power plug.

5　Weighing Method

Common weighing methods include direct weighing method, fixed mass weighing method and weight reduction weighing method.

5.1　Direct Weighing Method

Put the weighing object directly on the balance pan and directly weigh the mass of the object. For example, this method is used to weigh the small beaker, weigh the mass of a volumetric flask in the calibration of a volume vessel, and weigh the mass of a crucible in a gravimetric analysis experiment.

5.2　Fixed Mass Weighing Method

This method can also be called incremental method. It is used to weigh a fixed mass of reagent(such as a reference substance) or sample. The speed of this weighing method is very slow and it is suitable for weighing powder or small particles(minimum particles should be less than 0.1 mg in order to easily adjust the quality) of samples that are not easy to absorb moisture and can stably exist in the air.

When you use fixed mass weighing method, you should pay attention to the following operations:

If you accidentally add reagents that exceed the specified mass, use a spoon to remove excess reagents. Repeat the above operation until the quality of the reagent meets the specified requirements. Note that the removed excess reagents should be discarded and not returned to the original reagent bottle. The reagents cannot be scattered outside the container such as the balance plate during operation. The weighed reagents must be transferred directly from the container such as a weighing bottle to the receiving container quantitatively, that is, quantitative transfer.

The fixed mass weighing method is suitable for substances that are stable in air, do not absorb water, and do not react with oxygen, carbon dioxide and other substances. We can use containers such as weighing bottles and beakers.

5.3　Weight Reduction Weighing Method

This method can also be called decrement method. It can be used to weigh samples or reagents within a certain mass range. This method can be selected when the sample is easy to absorb water, easily oxidize or react with carbon dioxide during weighing. Since the quality of the weighed sample is obtained from the difference between the two weighings, it is also called subtraction method. Decrement methods are commonly used in drug analysis experiments, its operation procedure is as follows :

(1) Hold the weighing bottle with a paper tape from the dryer and remove the weighing bottle(you can also directly wear cotton, silicone or rubber gloves for operation), taking care not to let your fingers directly touch the bottle and bottle cap. Clamp and open the bottle

cap with a piece of paper, add an appropriate amount of sample(usually an integer multiple of the amount of a sample) with a drug spoon, and cap the bottle. Weigh out the exact mass of the weighing bottle with the sample.

（2）Remove the weighing bottle from the balance, tilt the bottle above the receiving container. Tap the upper part of the bottle mouth with the weighing bottle cap to slowly drop the sample into the container. The bottle cap should never leave above the receiving container. When the poured sample is closed to the required amount which can be estimated from the volume or the test weight, while it is continuing to tap the bottle mouth with the bottle cap, the bottle body is gradually straightened to make the the sample drop back into the weighing bottle. Then cover the bottle cap, accurately weigh the bottle.

（3）The difference between the two masses is the mass of the sample. Continuously decreasing according to the above method, multiple samples can be weighed. Sometimes it is difficult to obtain a sample that meets the quality range requirements at one time, the above weighing operation can be repeated 1 to 2 times.

6　Maintenance of Electronic Balance

The electronic balance room should avoid direct sunlight. It is best to choose a shaded room or take shading treatment. It should be far away from vibration sources, such as roads, shakers and other vibration machinery. When it is unavoidable, quakeproof measure should be taken. The electronic balance should be kept away from the environments with heat sources and high-intensity electromagnetic fields.

The temperature should be constant, preferably around 20 ℃, and the relative humidity in the work room should be 45% ～75%. The workroom should be clean and free of the influence of airflow and the corrosive gas.

Adjust the bubble of the balance level to the middle position before use. The electronic balance should be preheated according to the instructions. When weighing volatile and corrosive items, we should store the sample in a closed container to prevent corrosion and damage to the electronic balance. The electronic balance performs self-calibration or regular external calibration to ensure that it is in the best condition. If the electronic balance fails, it should be repaired in time, and it should not work with "illness". Do not overload the electronic balance to avoid damage to the balance.

7　Precautions for the Use of Balance

（1）Before opening the balance, check whether there are scattered materials on and around the balance weighing plate, and clean the inside of the weighing plate and balance box with a special balance brush. Lift the weighing plate vertically, check whether there is any scattered material, clean with a brush, put the weighing plate back carefully to its original position.

（2）Do not directly contact the chemical substances to be measured with the balance tray. Weigh in containers, such as weighing flasks, beakers, flasks or weighing paper, etc. , and try to use smaller containers for weighing.

（3）Place the sample to be weighed in the center of the weighing plate.

（4）When weighing objects, close the balance door to prevent air disturbance from interfering with the reading.

第三节　紫外－可见分光光度法

紫外－可见分光光度法是在 200～760 nm 波长范围内，通过测定被测物质在特定波长处或一定波长范围内对光的吸光度，对该物质进行定性和定量分析，如鉴别、杂质检查和含量测定。

常用的波长范围为 200～400 nm 的紫外光区，400～760 nm 的可见光区。所用仪器为紫外分光光度计、可见分光光度计（或比色计）。为保证测量的精密度和准确度，所用仪器应按照国家计量检定规程规定，定期进行校正检定。

单色光辐射穿过被测物质溶液时，在一定的浓度范围内被该物质吸收的量与该物质的浓度和液层的厚度（光路长度）成正比，符合朗伯－比尔定律，其关系式如下：

$$A = \lg \frac{1}{T} = ECL$$

式中，A 为吸光度；T 为透光率；E 为吸收系数，采用的表示方法是（$E_{cm}^{1\%}$），其物理意义为当溶液浓度为 1%（g/mL）、液层厚度为 1 cm 时的吸光度数值；C 为 100 mL 溶液中所含被测物质的重量（按干燥品或无水物计算），g；L 为液层厚度，cm。

物质对光的选择性吸收波长及相应的吸收系数是该物质的物理常数。当已知某纯物质在一定条件下的吸收系数后，可用同样条件将该供试品配成溶液，测定其吸收度，即可由上式计算出供试品中该物质的含量。在可见光区，除某些物质对光有吸收外，很多物质本身并没有吸收，但可在一定条件下加入显色试剂或经过处理使其显色后再测定，故又称比色分析。

一、仪器的校正和检定

（一）波长准确度

由于环境因素对机械部分的影响，仪器的波长经常会略有变动，因此，除应定期对所用的仪器进行全面校正检定外，还应于测定前校正测定波长。常用汞灯中的较强谱线如 237.83 nm、253.65 nm、275.28 nm、296.73 nm、313.16 nm、334.15 nm、365.02 nm、404.66 nm、435.83 nm、546.07 nm 与 576.96 nm 谱线，或用仪器中氘灯的 486.02 nm 与 656.10 nm 谱线进行校正，钬玻璃在 279.4 nm、287.5 nm、333.7 nm、360.9 nm、418.5 nm、460.0 nm、484.5 nm、536.2 nm 与 637.5 nm 波长

处有尖锐吸收峰，也可用作波长校正，但因来源不同或随着时间的推移会有微小的差别，使用时应注意。

波长的允许误差范围：紫外光区为 ±1 nm，500 nm 附近为 ±2 nm。

（二）吸光度的准确度

取在 120 ℃ 干燥至恒重的基准重铬酸钾约 60 mg，精密称定，用 0.005 mol/L 硫酸溶液溶解并稀释至 1 000 mL，在规定的波长处测定并计算其吸收系数，并与规定的吸收系数比较，应符合表 1-2-1 中的规定。

表 1-2-1　吸光度的准确度

波长/nm	235（最小）	257（最大）	313（最小）	350（最大）
吸收系数的规定值	124.5	144.0	48.62	106.6
吸收系数的许可范围	123.0～126.0	142.8～146.2	47.0～50.3	105.5～108.5

（三）杂散光的检查

按下表的试剂和浓度，配制成水溶液，置 1 cm 石英吸收池中，在规定的波长处测定透光率，应符合表 1-2-2 中的规定。

表 1-2-2　杂散光的检查

试剂	浓度/%（g/mL）	测定用波长/nm	透光率
碘化钠	1.00	220	<0.8%
亚硝酸钠	5.00	340	<0.8%

二、对溶剂要求

含有杂原子的有机溶剂，通常均具有很强的末端吸收。因此，当其作溶剂使用时，它们的使用范围均不能小于截止使用波长。例如，甲醇、乙醇的截止使用波长为 205 nm。另外，当溶剂不纯时，也可能增加干扰吸收。因此，在测定供试品前，应先检查所用的溶剂在供试品所用的波长附近是否符合要求，即将溶剂置 1 cm 石英吸收池中，以空气为空白（即空白光路中不置任何物质）测定其吸收度。溶剂和吸收池的吸光度，在 220～240 nm 范围内不得超过 0.40，在 241～250 nm 范围内不得超过 0.20，在 251～300 nm 范围内不得超过 0.10，在 300 nm 以上时不得超过 0.05。

进行测定时，除另有规定外，应以配制供试品溶液的同批溶剂为空白对照，采用 1 cm 的石英吸收池，在规定的吸收峰波长 ±2 nm 以内测试几个点的吸收度；或由仪器在规定波长附近自动扫描测定，以核对供试品的吸收峰波长位置是否正确，除另有规定外，吸收峰波长应在该品种项下规定的波长 ±2 nm 以内，并以吸光度最大的波长作为测定波长。一般供试品溶液的吸收度读数，以在 0.3～0.7 的误差较小。由于吸收池和溶剂本身可能有空白吸收，因此，测定供试品的吸光度后应减去空白读数，或由仪器自动扣除空白读数后再计算含量。

当溶液的 pH 对测定结果有影响时，应将供试品溶液和对照品溶液的 pH 调为一致。

三、含量测定

（一）对照品比较法

按各品种项下的方法，分别配制供试品溶液和对照品溶液，对照品溶液中所含被测成分的量应为供试品溶液中被测成分规定量的 100%±10%，所用溶剂也应完全一致，在规定的波长测定供试品溶液和对照品溶液的吸光度后，按下式计算供试品中被测溶液的浓度：

$$C_X = (A_X/A_R) C_R$$

式中，C_X 为供试品溶液的浓度，A_X 为供试品溶液吸收度，A_R 为对照品溶液的吸收度；C_R 为对照品溶液浓度。

（二）比色法

供试品溶液加入适量显色剂后测定吸光度以测定其含量的方法为比色法。用比色法测定时，应取数份梯度量的对照品溶液，用溶剂补充至同一体积，显色后，以相应试剂为空白，在各品种规定的波长处测定各份溶液的吸光度，以吸光度为纵坐标，浓度为横坐标绘制标准曲线，再根据供试品的吸光度在标准曲线上查得其相应的浓度，并求出其含量。也可取对照品溶液与供试品溶液同时操作，显色后，以相应的试剂为空白，在各品种规定的波长处测定对照品和供试品溶液的吸光度，按上述对照品比较法计算供试品溶液的浓度。除另有规定外，比色法所用空白系指用同体积溶剂代替对照品或供试品溶液，然后依次加入等量的相应试剂，并用同样方法处理制得。

（三）吸收系数法

按各品种项下的方法配制供试品溶液，测定其在规定波长下的吸光度，在规定条件下，按规定的吸收系数计算其含量：

$$C_X = A/(E_{cm}^{1\%} \cdot L)$$

式中，C_X 为供试品溶液的浓度；A 为供试品溶液的吸光度；$E_{cm}^{1\%}$ 为产品在规定条件下的吸收系数；L 为液层厚度，cm。

Section 3　Ultraviolet Visible Spectrophotometry

Ultraviolet visible spectrophotometry is a method to measure the absorbance of light between the wavelengths of 200 nm and 760 nm by substances for qualitative and quantitative analysis of the substance at a specific wavelength or within a certain wavelength range, such as identification, impurity inspection and content determination.

The commonly used wavelength ranges are divided into the ultraviolet region($200 \sim 400$ nm) and visible region ($400 \sim 760$ nm) . The instruments used are ultraviolet spectrophotometer, visible spectrophotometer(or colorimeter). In order to ensure the precision and accuracy of measurement, the instruments used should be calibrated regularly according to the national metrological verification regulations.

When monochromatic light radiation passes through the measured substance solution, the amount absorbed by the substance within a certain concentration range is directly proportional to the concentration of the substance and the thickness(optical path length) of the liquid layer, this relation is expressed by the Lamber-Beer's law with the following equation:

$$A = \lg \frac{1}{T} = ECL$$

where A is the absorbance; T is the transmittance; E is the absorption coefficient, which is expressed by($E_{cm}^{1\%}$) ; The term denote the absorbance of a 1% solution in a 1 cm cell. C is the concentration of the substance expressed in g per 100 mL solution, calculated on the dried or dehydrated basis; L is absorption path length expressed in cm.

The selective absorption wavelength and the corresponding absorption coefficient are the physical constants of a substance. When the absorption coefficient of a pure substance under certain conditions is known, the test substance can be prepared into a solution under the same conditions, and its absorbance can be determined, then the content of the substance in the test substance can be calculated from the above formula. In the visible light region, except some substances have absorption of light, many substances themselves have no absorption, but they can be determined after adding color reagent or treatment under certain conditions, so it is also called colorimetric analysis.

1　Calibration and Verification of Instruments

1. 1　Wavelength Accuracy

The influence of environmental factors on the mechanical part of the spectrophotometer and cause a drift of the wavelength scale slightly, therefore, the spectrophotometer should be calibrated regularly, and the wavelength scale should be verified before the measurement. The stronger spectral lines of 237. 83 nm, 253. 65 nm, 275. 28 nm, 296. 73 nm, 313. 16 nm, 334. 15 nm, 365. 02 nm, 404. 66 nm, 435. 83 nm, 546. 07 nm and 576. 96 nm from the mercury lamp are common used, or 486. 02 nm and 656. 10 nm from the deuterium lamp are used for calibration. There are sharp absorption peaks at 279. 4 nm, 287. 5 nm, 333. 7 nm, 360. 9 nm, 418. 5 nm, 460. 0 nm, 484. 5 nm, 536. 2 nm and 637. 5 nm in holmium glass, which also can be used for wavelength calibration, but there will be slight differences due to different light sources or along with the time going by, we should pay attention to it.

The permitted tolerance of the the instrument wavelength is ± 1 nm for the ultraviolet region and ± 2 nm nearby 500 nm.

1. 2 Accuracy of Absorbance

Take about 60 mg of standard potassium dichromate dried at 120 ℃ to constant weight, accurately weigh, dissolve it with 0. 005 mol/L sulfuric acid solution and dilute it to 1 000 mL, measure and calculate its absorption coefficient at the specified wavelength, and compare it with the specified absorption coefficient, which shall meet the requirements in Tab. 1 − 2 − 1.

Tab 1 −2 −1   Accuracy of absorbance

Wavelength/nm	235(min)	257(max)	313(min)	350(max)
Specific absorbance	124. 5	144. 0	48. 62	106. 6
Maximum	123. 0 ～ 126. 0	142. 8 ～ 146. 2	47. 0 ～ 50. 3	105. 5 ～ 108. 5

1. 3 Check of Stray Light

The reagent and concentration in the following table shall be prepared with an aqueous solution and placed into a 1 cm quartz absorption cell. The light transmittance shall be determined at the specified wavelength, which shall meet the requirements in Tab. 1 − 2 − 2.

Tab 1 −2 −2   The check of stray light

Reagent	Concentration/% (g/mL)	Wavelength /nm	Transmittance
Sodium iodide	1. 00	220	<0. 8%
Sodium nitrite	5. 00	340	<0. 8%

2 Requirements for the Solvents

The organic solvents containing heteroatoms usually have strong terminal absorption. Therefore, when they are used as solvents, their application range should be greater than the cut-off wavelength. For example, the cut-off wavelength of methanol and ethanol is 205 nm. In addition, when the solvent is impure, the interference absorption may also be increased. Therefore, before determining the sample, it is necessary to check whether the solvent used meets the requirements near the wavelength used by the sample, that is, the solvent is placed in a 1 cm quartz absorption cell, and the air is used as the blank(that is, no matter is placed in the empty white light path) to determine its absorbance. The absorbance of solvent and absorption cell shall not exceed 0. 40 in the range of 220 nm to 240 nm, 0. 20 in the range of 241 nm to 250 nm, 0. 10 in the range of 251 nm to 300 nm, and 0. 05 at the wavelengths above 300 nm.

Unless otherwise specified, the same batch of solvent used to prepare the test solution shall be used as blank control, and the absorptivity of several points shall be tested within ± 2 nm of the specified absorption peak wavelength in a 1 cm quartz absorption cell, or the instrument shall scan and measure automatically near the specified wavelength to check whether the wavelength of the maximum absorption of the test sample is correct. Unless otherwise specified, the wavelength of absorption maximum shall be within ± 2 nm of the specified wavelength, the assay should be carry out at the wavelength of the maximum absorption.

Generally, the absorbance reading for the test solution has a smaller error between 0. 3 to 0. 7, because there may be blank absorption in the absorption cell and the solvent itself, the blank reading should be subtracted after determining the absorbance of the test sample, or the content should be calculated after the blank reading is automatically deducted by the instrument.

When the pH value of the solution has influence on the determination results, the pH value of the test solution should be adjusted to be equal to that of the reference solution.

3 The Methods for Content Determination

3. 1 Reference Substance Comparison Method

Prepare the test solution and the reference solution separately according to the method under item of the individual monograph. The content of the tested component in the reference solution shall be 100% ± 10% of the labelled amount of the tested component in the test solution, and the solvents used shall be completely consistent. After the absorbance of the test solution and the reference substance solution is determined at the specified wavelength, the concentration of the compound in the test solution shall be calculated according to the following formula:

$$C_X = (A_X/A_R) C_R$$

where C_X is the concentration of the test solution; A_X is the absorbance of the test solution; A_R is the absorbance of the reference substance solution; C_R is the concentration of the the reference substance solution.

3. 2 Colorimetry

The colorimetric method is used to determine the content of the test sample solution by measuring the absorbance after adding an appropriate amount of chromogenic agent. When colorimetric method is used for determination, several parts of gradient reference solution shall be taken and added to the same volume with solvent. After color development, the absorbance of each solution shall be determined at the wavelength under the specified monograph with corresponding reagent as blank. The standard curve shall be drawn with the absorbance as ordinate and the concentration as abscissa, and then the corresponding concentration shall be found on the standard curve according to the absorbance of the test sample, and the corresponding concentration shall be determined, then its content is determined. It is also advisable to determine the reference solution and the test solution at the same time. After color development, the absorbance of the reference solution and the test solution can be determined at the specified wavelength under the specified monograph with the corresponding reagent as blank. The concentration of the test solution can be calculated according to the above method 3. 1. Unless otherwise specified, the blank used in colorimetry refers to replace the reference solution or the test solution with the same volume of solvent, and then adding it in turn.

3. 3 Absorption Coefficient Method

Prepare the solution of the substance being examined according to the method under the specified monograph, measure its absorption at the specified wavelength, and then calculate the content according to the absorption coefficient specified in the monograph under the specified conditions as follows:

$$C_X = A / (E_{cm}^{1\%} \cdot L)$$

where C_X is the concentration of the test solution; A is the absorbance of the test solution; $E_{cm}^{1\%}$ is the absorption coefficient of the product under the specified conditions; L is the thickness of the liquid layer, in cm.

第四节　薄层色谱法

薄层色谱法（thin later chromatography，TLC）是指将供试品溶液点于薄层板上，在展开容器内用展开剂展开，使供试品所含成分分离，所得色谱图与适宜的对照物按同法所得的色谱图对比，并可用薄层扫描仪进行扫描，用于鉴别、检查或含量测定。

一、仪器与材料

（一）薄层板

市售薄层板分普通薄层板和高效薄层板两种，如硅胶薄层板、硅胶 GF$_{254}$薄层板、化学键合硅胶薄层板、聚酰胺薄膜等。

自制薄层板在保证色谱质量的前提下，若需要对薄层板进行特别处理和化学改性以适应供试品分离的要求时，也可用实验室自制的薄层板。最常用的固定相有硅胶 G、硅胶 GF$_{254}$、硅胶 H、硅胶 HF$_{254}$、微晶纤维素等，其颗粒大小一般要求直径为 10～40 μm，加水或用羧甲基纤维素钠水溶液（0.2%～0.5%）适量调成糊状，均匀涂布于玻板上。涂布时应能使固定相在玻板上涂成一层符合厚度要求的均匀薄层。玻璃板应光滑、平整，洗净后不附水珠。

（二）点样器

点样器一般采用微量注射器、微升毛细管，或手动、半自动、全自动点样器材。

（三）展开容器

上行展开一般可用适合薄层板大小的专用平底或有双槽的展开缸，展开时须能密闭，水平展开用专用的水平展开缸。

（四）显色装置

喷雾显色应使用玻璃喷雾瓶或专用喷雾器，用压缩气体使显色剂呈均匀细雾状喷出；浸渍显色可用专用玻璃器械或用适宜的展开缸代替；蒸气熏蒸显色可用双槽展开缸或适宜大小的干燥器代替。

（五）检视装置

检视装置有可见光、254 nm 和 365 nm 紫外光光源及相应的滤光片的暗箱，可附加摄像设备供拍摄图像用，暗箱内光源应有足够的光照度。

（六）薄层色谱扫描仪

薄层色谱扫描仪系指用一定波长的光对薄层板上有吸收的斑点或经激发后能发射出荧光的斑点进行扫描，将扫描得到的谱图和积分数据用于物质定性或定量的分析仪器。

二、操作方法

（一）薄层板制备

市售薄层板临用前一般应在 110 ℃活化 30 min，置干燥器中备用。聚酰胺薄膜不需要活化。铝基片薄层板可根据需要剪裁，但须注意剪裁后的薄层板底边的硅胶层不得有破损。除另有规定外，将 1 份固定相和 3 份水（或加有黏合剂的水溶液）在研钵中按同一方向研磨混合，去除表面的气泡后，倒入涂布器中，在玻璃板上平稳地移动涂布器进行涂布（厚度为 0.2～0.3 mm），取下涂好薄层的玻璃板，置水平台上于室温下晾干后，在 110 ℃烘 30 min，置有干燥剂的干燥箱中备用。使用前检查其均匀度，在反射光及透视光下检视，其表面应均匀、平整、光滑，无麻点、无气泡、无破损及污染。

（二）点样

除另有规定外，在洁净干燥的环境，用专用毛细管或配合相应的半自动、自动点样器械点样于薄层板上，一般为圆点状或窄细的条带状，点样基线距底边 10～15 mm，高效板基线一般离底边 8～10 mm。圆点状直径一般不大于 3 mm，高效板一般不大于

2 mm；接触点样时注意勿损伤薄层表面。条带状宽度一般为 5～10 mm。高效板条带宽度一般为 4～8 mm，可用专用半自动或自动点样器械喷雾法点样。点间距离可视斑点扩散情况以相邻斑点互不干扰为宜，一般不少于 8 mm，高效板供试品间隔不少于 5 mm。

（三）展开

将点好样品的薄层板放入展开缸的展开剂中，浸入展开剂的深度为距原点 5 mm 为宜，密闭。除另有规定外，一般上行展开 8～15 cm，高效薄层板上展开 5～8 cm。溶剂前沿达到规定的展距，取出薄层板，晾干，待检测。

展开前若需要溶剂蒸气预平衡，可在展开缸中加入适量的展开剂，密闭，一般保持 15～30 min。溶剂蒸气预平衡后，应迅速放入载有供试品的薄层板，立即密闭，展开。若需要使展开缸达到溶剂蒸汽饱和的状态，则须在展开缸的内侧放置与展开缸内径同样大小的滤纸，密闭一定时间，使达到饱和再如法展开。必要时，可进行二次展开或双向展开。

（四）显色与检视

供试品含有可见光下有颜色的成分时可直接在日光下检视，也可用喷雾法或浸渍法以适宜的显色剂显色，或加热显色，在日光下检视。有荧光的物质或遇某些试剂可激发荧光的物质可在 365 nm 或 254 nm 紫外光灯下观察其荧光色谱。对于可见光下无色，但在紫外光下有吸收的成分可用带有荧光剂的硅胶板（如硅胶 GF_{254} 板），在 254 nm 紫外光灯下观察荧光板面上的荧光猝灭物质形成的色谱。

（五）记录

薄层色谱图像一般可采用摄像设备拍摄，以光学照片或电子图像的形式保存。也可用薄层扫描仪扫描记录相应的色谱图。

三、系统适用性试验

按各品种项下要求对实验条件进行系统适用性试验，即用供试品和对照品对实验条件进行试验和调整，应达到规定的检测灵敏度、分离度和重复性要求。

（一）比移值

比移值（R_f）系指从基线至展开斑点中心的距离与从基线至展开剂前沿的距离的比值：其计算公式为

$$R_f = \frac{基线至展开斑点中心的距离}{基线至展开剂前沿的距离}$$

除另有规定外，杂质检查时，杂质斑点的 R_f 以 0.2～0.8 为宜。

（二）检出限

用于限量检查时，供试品溶液、对照品溶液与稀释若干倍的对照品溶液在规定的色谱条件下，于同一薄层板上点样、展开、检视，后者应显清晰的斑点。此浓度或量作为检出限。

（三）分离度

用于鉴别时，对照品溶液与供试品溶液中相应的主斑点，应显示2个清晰分离的斑点。用于限量检查和含量测定时，要求定量峰与相邻峰之间有较好的分离度（R）。其计算公式为

$$R = \frac{2(d_2 - d_1)}{(W_1 + W_2)}$$

式中，d_2 为相邻两峰中后一峰与原点的距离，d_1 为相邻两峰中前一峰与原点的距离，W_1 及 W_2 为相邻两峰各自的峰宽。除另有规定外，分离度应大于1.0。

（四）重复性

同一供试品溶液在同一薄层板上平行点样的待测成分的峰面积测量值的相对标准偏差应不大于3.0%；需要显色后测定的相对标准偏差应不大于5.0%。

四、测定法

（一）鉴别

取适宜浓度的对照溶液与供试品溶液，在同一薄层板上点样、展开与检视，供试品溶液所显主斑点的颜色（或荧光）和位置应与对照溶液的斑点一致。

（二）限量检查

采用定量配制的对照品对照或对照品稀释液对照。供试品溶液色谱中待检查的斑点与相应的对照品溶液或系列对照品溶液的相应斑点比较，颜色（或荧光）不得更深；或按照薄层色谱扫描法操作，供试品的峰面积不得大于对照品的峰面积值。必要时应规定检查的斑点数和限量值。

（三）含量测定

按照薄层色谱扫描法，测定供试品中相应成分的含量。

五、薄层色谱扫描法

薄层色谱扫描法是指用一定波长的光照射在薄层板上，对薄层色谱中可吸收紫外光或可见光的斑点，或经激发后能发射出荧光的斑点进行扫描，将扫描得到的图谱及积分数据用于药品的鉴别、检查或含量测定。测定时可根据不同薄层扫描仪的结构特点，按照规定方式扫描测定，一般选择反射方式，采用吸收法或荧光法。除另有规定外，含量测定应使用市售薄层板。

扫描方法可采用单波长扫描或双波长扫描。若采用双波长扫描，应选用待测斑点无吸收或最小吸收的波长为参比波长，供试品色谱中待测斑点的比移值（R_f）和光谱扫描得到的吸收光谱图或测得的光谱最大吸收与最小吸收应与对照品相符，以保证测定结果的准确性。薄层扫描定量测定应保证供试品斑点的量在线性范围内，必要时可适当调整供试品溶液的点样量，供试品与对照品同板点样、展开、扫描、测定和

计算。

薄层色谱扫描用于含量测定时，通常采用线性回归二点法计算，当线性范围很窄时，可用多点法校正多项式回归计算。供试品溶液和对照品溶液应交叉点于同一薄层板上，供试品点样不得少于2个，对照品每一浓度点样不得少于2个。扫描时，应沿展开方向扫描，不可横向扫描。

Section 4　Thin Layer Chromatography(TLC)

The thin layer chromatography(TLC) is a separation method in which the test solutions are deposited on the thin layer plate and developed by the mobile phase in a chromatographic chamber to separate the components of the substance being examined. The chromatogram obtained is compared with that of the appropriate reference substances under the same conditions and can be scanned by the TLC scanning instrument. The results can be used for identification, inspection or content determination.

1　Instruments and Materials

1.1　Thin Layer Plate

The marketed thin layer plates are divided into ordinary thin layer plates and high-efficiency thin layer plates, such as silica gel thin layer plates, silica gel GF_{254} thin layer plates, chemical bonded silica gel thin layer plates, polyamide film, etc.

On the premise of ensuring the quality of chromatography, if special treatment and chemical modification are needed to meet the separation requirements of the test sample, the self-made thin-layer plate can also be used. The most commonly used stationary phases are silica gel G, silica gel GF_{254}, silica gel H, silica gel HF_{254}, microcrystalline cellulose, etc. The particle size of the stationary phase is generally required to be $10 \sim 40$ μm in diameter. Add water or use sodium carboxymethyl cellulose aqueous solution ($0.2\% \sim 0.5\%$)to make a paste and evenly spread on the glass plate. When coating, the stationary phase shall be coated on the glass plate into a uniform thin layer to meet the thickness requirements. The glass plate shall be smooth and flat, and there shall be no water drop after cleaning.

1.2　Sample Applicator

The microsyringe, micro liter capillary or manual, semi-automatic and full-automatic applicator are generally used for the sampling device.

1.3　Chromatographic Chamber

The special flat bottomed or double grooved developing cylinder suitable for the size of thin plate can be used for the upward developing. The chamber must be airtight, and the special horizontal cylinder can be used for the horizontal developing.

1. 4　Visualization Device

The glass spray bottle or special sprayer can be used for atomizing develop. Compressed gas can be used to eject the visualization reagent in the form of homogeneous mist. Special glass apparatus or appropriate glass chamber can be used instead during the immersion visualization. Double trough glass chamber or desiccator with appropriately size could be used during the fumigation visualization.

1. 5　Detection Device

The dark box with visible light, 254 nm and 365 nm ultraviolet light sources and corresponding filters can be attached with camera equipment for image shooting. The light resource in the dark box should have enough intensity of illumination.

1. 6　Thin Layer Chromatography Scanner

It is used to scan the spots, which can absorb the light of certain wavelength or emit fluorescence after being excited. The obtained scanning profiles of the chromatogram and the integration data can be used for qualitative or quantitative analysis of substances.

2　Procedure

2. 1　Preparation of Thin Layer Plates

The commercial thin layer plate should be activated at 110 ℃ for 30 min before use, and put it into the dryer for future use. Polyamide film does not need activation. Aluminum thin plate can be cut according to the needs, but the silica gel layer at the bottom of the cut thin plate must not be damaged.

Unless otherwise specified, grind and mix one part of stationary phase and three parts of water(or aqueous solution with adhesive) in the mortar in one direction, remove the bubbles on the surface, pour them into the spreader, move the spreader smoothly on the glass plate for coating(the thickness is 0. 2 ～ 0. 3 mm) , remove the coated glass plate, allow the plate to be dried on a horizontal plane at the room temperature. Heat it at 110 ℃ for 30 min, and then store it in a desiccator for later use. Check the degree of the homogeneity under both the reflected light and the transmitted light. The surface of the plate should be uniform, flat, smooth, without rough portion, bubble, breakage or contamination.

2. 2　Sample Application

Unless otherwise specified, the samples are applied on the TLC plates, usually in the form of circular spots or narrow bands, with special capillary or semi-automatic and automatic sample applicators under a clean and dry environment. The distance of the sample zone from the lower edge of TLC plate is 10 ～ 15 mm, while that of HPTLC plates is 8 ～ 10 mm. The diameter of the circular pots is generally not more than 3 mm for TLC, while not more than 2 mm for HPTLC. Pay attention do not damage the surface of the thin-layer where the sample applied. The width of the bands is generally 5 ～ 10 mm for TLC, while 4 ～ 8 mm for

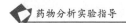

HPTLC. Sample could also be applied by spraying method with special semi-automatic or automatic sample applicators. Spots intervals should be adjusted according to the diffusion of the spots and with no interference between neighboring spots. Usually, the interval is not less than 8 mm for TLC, not less than 5 mm for HPTLC.

2.3 Development

Place the plate loaded with sample into the chromatographic chamber, keeping a distance of about 5 mm from the line of applying sample to the edge of solvent specified, for ascending development, usually $8 \sim 15$ cm will be developed for TLC, while $5 \sim 8$ cm for HPTLC. When the mobile phase has moved over the prescribed development distance, remove the plate from the chamber, mark the mobile phase front and dry it for later detection.

If the chamber should be pre-equilibrated before development, add appropriate amount of mobile phase into the chromatographic chamber. Close the chamber tightly and usually maintain for $15 \sim 30$ min. After the vapor of solvent has reach equilibrium, place the plate loaded with samples quickly into the chamber and close it immediately tightly for development. If the vapor of the solvent should be saturated in the chromatographic chamber, filter paper of the same dimension with the inner diameter of the chamber should be laid on the inner wall of the chamber and one end of the filter paper is immersed into the mobile phase. Keep the chamber tightly for a while and allow it to be fully saturated before developing.

If necessary, secondary development and two-dimension development could be applied. The residual mobile phase on the thin-layer plates should be evaporated before the second development.

2.4 Visualization and Detection

The coloured substances could be detected directly under visible light. The colourless substances may be visualized with appropriate visualization reagent by the way of spraying or immersion. They could also be visualized by being heated and detected directly under the visible light. The fluorescence spots of the fluorescent substances or the substances which may excite fluorescence may be visualized under the UV lamp(365 nm or 254 nm). The silica gel plates containing fluorescence(such as silica gel GF_{254} plates) could be used if the components have ultraviolet absorption. The spots formed by the quenching of fluorescent substance on the plate can be observed under the UV lamp(254 nm).

2.5 Documentation

The image of the TLC could be taken by camera and saved in the form of optical picture or electronic image. The TLC scanning instrument and other suitable method could also record the corresponding chromatogram.

3 System Suitability Test

The system suitability test should be carried out for the experiment conditions according to the requirements specified under the monograph. The test solution and the reference solution are used to test and adjust the experiment condition in order to meet the prescribed requirements.

3. 1　The Retardation Factor(R_f)

It is defined as the ratio of the distance from the point of application to the center of the spot and the distance from the point of application to the mobile phase front.

R_f = the distance from the point of application to the center of the spot/the distance from the point of application to the mobile phase front.

Unless otherwise specified, when impurities are tested, for spots of impurities, the retardation factor(R_f) should be controlled within 0. 2 ～ 0. 8.

3. 2　Detection Limit

It is the minimum concentration or amount of the substance being examined which can be detected in the test solution in limit test or impurity test. Usually the test solution or reference standard solution with known concentrations, and series dilute self-control reference standard solution are applied, developed and visualized on the same TLC plate under the prescribed chromatograph conditions. The concentration or amount of the reference standard solution when clear and distinguishable spot is exhibited is the detection limit.

3. 3　Resolution

For identification testing, the main spot(s) in the reference solution and in the test solution should be clearly separated. For limit test or assay, the peak used for quantification should be well separated with the adjacent peak. The formula for calculating the resolution(R) is

$$R = \frac{2(d_2 - d_1)}{(W_1 + W_2)}$$

where d_2 is the distance between the latter of the two adjacent peaks and the original point; d_1 is the distance between the former of the two adjacent peaks and the original; W_2 and W_1 is the peak width of the two adjacent point peaks respectively.

Unless otherwise specified, the resolution should be more than 1. 0.

3. 4　Repeatability

When the same test solution is applied in parallel on the same thin-layer plate, the relative standard deviation of the peak areas of the ingredients being examined should be not more than 3. 0%. The relative standard deviation for those which should be determined after visualization or on different plates should be not more than 5. 0%.

4　Measurement

4. 1　Identification

The reference solution and the test solution of appropriate concentration are prepared, applied, developed and visualized on the same TLC plate with the method prescribed under the monograph. The colour(or fluorescence) and the position of the main spot(s) of the test solution should be identical with those of the spot(s) of the reference solution.

4.2 Limit Test

The reference solution and the test solution of appropriate concentration are prepared. The colour(or fluorescence) of the spot being examined in the chromatogram of the test solution should be not more intense compared to the corresponding spot of the reference solution. Or, the peak area may be determined according to the method of TLC scanning and the peak area of the corresponding spot in the chromatogram of the test solution should be not more than the peak area of the reference solution. If it is necessary, the number of spots and limit value should be specified.

4.3 Assay

According to the TLC scanning method, the content of the corresponding components in the test sample is determined.

5 TLC Scanning Method

It is to scan the spots, which can absorb ultraviolet light or visible light or which can emit fluorescens after being excited, exposing the TLC plate light of a certain wavelength. Thus obtained chromatograms and integral data are used to identify, test or assay. According to the structural characteristics of different scanning instrument, the spots may be scanned and determined based on specified method. Generally, reflective scanning mode in the absorbance method or fluorescence method is frequently used. Unless otherwise specified, the commercial pre-coated TLC plates should be used in the assay.

Single-wavelength scanning or dual-wavelength scanning method could be used. For dual-wavelength scanning, the wavelength at which the spots being examined have no absorption or the minimum absorption should be used as a reference wavelength. In the chromatogram of the test solution, the retardation factor(R_f) of the spots being examined the absorption spectrum obtained from the spectrum scanning or the obtained maximum absorption an minimum absorption of the spectrum should be identical with those of the reference solution to ensure the accuracy of determination results. For the quantitative analysis by using the TLC scanning method, it should be ensured that the amount of the spot being examined is within the linear range. If necessary, the amount of the test solution being applied or the plate could be adjusted appropriately. The test solution could be applied, developed, scanned, measured and calculated on the same plate with the reference solution.

When the TLC scanning method is used for assay, linear regression two-point method is usually adopted for calculation. If the linear range is very narrow, multinomial regression of multiple level of standard calibration could be used. The test solution and the reference solution should be applied alternatively on the same TLC plate. The number of the spots of the test solution should not be less than 2 and that of the reference solution should not be less than 2 for each concentration. Scan the plate along the direction of development, but not horizontally.

第五节　高效液相色谱法

高效液相色谱法系采用高压输液泵将规定的流动相泵入装有填充剂的色谱柱，对供试品进行分离测定的色谱方法。注入的供试品，由流动相带入色谱柱内，各组分在柱内被分离，并进入检测器检测，由积分仪或数据处理系统记录和处理色谱信号。高效液相色谱仪分析流程见图 1 - 2 - 1。

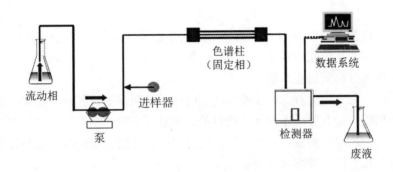

图 1 - 2 - 1　高效液相色谱仪分析流程

一、对仪器的一般要求与色谱条件

高效液相色谱仪由高压输液泵、进样器、色谱柱、检测器、积分仪或数据处理系统组成。色谱柱内径一般为 3.9～4.6 mm，填充剂粒径为 3～10 μm。超高效液相色谱仪是使用小粒径（约 2 μm）填充剂的耐超高压、小进样量、低死体积、高灵敏度检测的高效液相色谱仪。

（一）色谱柱

1. 反相色谱柱

反相色谱柱是以键合非极性基团的载体为填充剂填充而成的色谱柱。常见的载体有硅胶、聚合物复合硅胶和聚合物等；常用的填充剂有十八烷基硅烷键合硅胶（C_{18}）、辛基硅烷键合硅胶（C_8）和苯基硅烷键合硅胶等。

2. 正相色谱柱

正相色谱柱是用硅胶填充剂或键合极性基团的硅胶填充而成的色谱柱。常见的填充剂有硅胶、氨基键合硅胶和氰基键合硅胶等。这三种正向柱也都可用作反相色谱。

3. 离子交换色谱柱

离子交换色谱柱是用离子交换填充剂填充而成的色谱柱。其有阳离子交换色谱柱和阴离子交换色谱柱。

4. 手性分离色谱柱

手性分离色谱柱是用手性填充剂填充而成的色谱柱，用于分离手性化合物。

色谱柱的内径与长度、填充剂的形状、载体表面基团残留量、粒径与粒径分布、表面积、孔径、键合基团的表面覆盖度、填充的致密与均匀程度等均影响色谱柱的性能，应根据被分离物质的性质来选择合适的色谱柱。

温度会影响分离效果，未指明色谱柱温度时系指室温（10 ～ 30 ℃），应注意室温变化的影响。为改善分离效果可适当提高色谱柱的温度，但最好不要超过 60 ℃。

残余硅羟基未封闭的硅胶色谱柱，适用的流动相 pH 一般应为 2 ～ 8。烷基硅烷带有立体侧链保护、残余硅羟基已封闭的硅胶、聚合物复合硅胶或聚合物色谱柱可耐受更广泛 pH 的流动相，可用于 pH 小于 2 或大于 8 的流动相。

（二）检测器

最常用的检测器（detector）为紫外－可见分光检测器，包括二极管阵列检测器，其他常见的检测器有荧光检测器、蒸发光散射检测器、电喷雾检测器、示差折光检测器、电化学检测器和质谱检测器等。

紫外－可见分光检测器、荧光检测器、电化学检测器为选择性检测器，其响应值不仅与被测物质的量有关，还与其结构有关；蒸发光散射检测器、电喷雾检测器和示差折光检测器为通用检测器，对所有物质均有响应，结构相似的物质在蒸发光散射检测器的响应值几乎仅与被测物质的量有关。

紫外－可见分光检测器、荧光检测器、电化学检测器和示差折光检测器的响应值与被测物质的量在一定范围内符合朗伯－比尔定律，呈线性关系；蒸发光散射检测器的响应值与被测物质的量通常呈指数关系，一般需要经对数转换；电喷雾检测器的响应值与被测物质的量通常也呈指数关系，一般需要经对数转换或用二次函数计算，但在小质量范围内可基本呈线性。

不同的检测器，对流动相的要求不同。紫外－可见分光检测器所用流动相应符合紫外－可见分光光度法［《中国药典（2020 年版）》通则 0401］项下对溶剂的要求；采用低波长检测时，还应考虑有机溶剂的截止使用波长，并选用色谱级有机溶剂。蒸发光散射检测器、电喷雾检测器和质谱检测器不得使用含不挥发性成分的流动相。

（三）流动相

反相色谱系统的流动相（mobile phase）常用甲醇—水系统或乙腈—水系统，用紫外末端波长检测时，宜选用乙腈—水系统。流动相中应尽可能不用缓冲盐，若需要用时，应尽可能使用低浓度缓冲盐。用十八烷基硅烷键合硅胶色谱柱时，流动相中有机溶剂一般应不低于 5%，否则易导致柱效下降、色谱系统不稳定；或采用内嵌极性基团键合固定相色谱柱。

正相色谱系统的流动相常用两种或两种以上的有机溶剂，如二氯甲烷和正己烷等。

流动相的洗脱方式分为等度洗脱和梯度洗脱两种。用梯度洗脱分离时，梯度洗脱程序可以表格形式呈现，其中包括运行时间和流动相在不同时间的成分比例。

（四）色谱参数调整

质量标准中品种正文项下规定的色谱条件，除填充剂种类、检测器类型、流动相组分不得改变外，其余如色谱柱内径与长度、填充剂粒径、流动相组分比例、流动相流速、柱温、进样量、检测器灵敏度等，均可适当调整，以达到系统适用性试验的要求。调整流动相组分比例时，当小比例组分的百分比例 X 小于等于33%，允许改变范围为 $0.7X \sim 1.3X$；当 X 大于33%，允许改变范围为 $0.9X \sim 1.1X$。

若需要使用小粒径（约2 μm）填充剂以提高分离度或缩短分析时间，输液泵的性能、进样体积、检测池体积和系统的死体积等必须与之匹配，若有必要，色谱条件（参数）可适当调整。

色谱参数允许调整范围见表1-2-3。

表1-2-3 色谱柱、填料粒径和相应参数允许调整的范围

参数变量	参数调整
固定相	不能改变固定相的理化性质，如填料材质、表面修饰及键合相均需要保持一致。在满足上述条件的前提下，允许由全孔填料改为表面孔填料
填料粒径（dp），柱长（L）	改变色谱柱粒径和柱长后，L/dp 值（或 N 值）应为原有数值的 $-25\% \sim +50\%$
流速	可以根据实际使用时系统压力和保留时间，允许流速在 $\pm50\%$ 的范围内进行调整
进样体积	根据灵敏度的需求进行调整。即便未对色谱柱尺寸进行调整，进样体积也可调整以满足系统适用性的要求
梯度洗脱程序（不适用等度洗脱）	保持不同规格色谱柱的洗脱体积倍数相同，从而保证梯度变化相同，并需要考虑不同仪器系统体积的差异
等度洗脱流动相比例（不适于梯度洗脱）	最小比例的流动相组分可在相对值 $\pm30\%$ 或者绝对值 $\pm2\%$ 的范围内进行调整（两者之间选择最大值）；最小比例流动相组分的比例应小于 $(100/n)\%$，n 为流动相中组分的个数
流动相缓冲液盐浓度	可在 $\pm10\%$ 范围内调整
柱温	当温度有规定时，可在 $\pm10℃$ 范围内调整
pH	除另有规定外，流动相中水相 pH 可在 ±0.2pH 范围内进行调整
检测波长	不允许改变

表1-2-3中进样量、流速和梯度洗脱程序的调整范围可通过相关软件计算，并根据色谱峰的分离情况进行微调。应评价色谱参数调整对分离和检测的影响，若调整超出表1-2-3中规定的范围，对调整的方法应进行相应的方法学验证。调整后，系统适用性应符合要求，且色谱峰出峰顺序不变。若减小进样体积，应保证检测限和峰

面积的重复性；若增加进样体积，应使分离度和线性关系仍满足要求。

对于梯度洗脱，如调整梯度洗脱色谱参数应比调整等度洗脱色谱参数更加谨慎，因为此调整可能会使某些峰位置变化，造成峰识别错误，或者与其他峰合并。

无论调整后的方法验证与否，当对调整色谱条件后的测定结果产生异议时，应以品种项下规定的色谱条件的测定结果为准。

在品种项下一般不宜指定或推荐色谱柱的品牌，但可规定色谱柱的填料（固定相）种类（如键合相，是否改性、封端等）、粒径、孔径，色谱柱的柱长或柱内径；当耐用性试验证明必须使用特定牌号的色谱柱方能满足分离要求时，可在该品种正文项下注明。

二、系统适用性试验

色谱系统的适用性试验通常包括分离度、理论板数、灵敏度、拖尾因子和重复性5个参数。

按各标准项下要求对色谱系统进行适用性试验，即用规定的对照品溶液或系统适用性试验溶液在规定的色谱系统进行试验，必要时，可对色谱系统进行适当调整，以符合要求。

（一）色谱柱的理论板数

色谱柱的理论板数（n）用于评价色谱柱的效能。由于不同物质在同一色谱柱上的色谱行为不同，采用理论板数作为衡量色谱柱效能的指标时，应指明测定物质，一般为待测物质或内标物质的理论板数。

在规定的色谱条件下，注入供试品溶液或各品种项下规定的内标物质溶液，记录色谱图。测量出供试品主成分色谱峰或内标物质色谱峰的保留时间（t_R）和峰宽（W）或半高峰宽（$W_{h/2}$），按 $n = 16 \ (t_R/W)^2$ 或 $n = 5.54 \ (t_R/W_{h/2})^2$ 计算色谱柱的理论板数。t_R、W、$W_{h/2}$ 可用时间或长度计（下同），但应取相同单位。

（二）分离度

分离度（R）用于评价待测物质与被分离物质之间的分离程度，是衡量色谱系统分离效能的关键指标。可以通过测定待测物质与已知杂质的分离度，或通过测定待测物质与某一指标性成分（内标物质或其他难分离物质）的分离度，或将供试品/对照品用适当的方法降解后通过测定待测物质与某一降解产物的分离度，对色谱系统分离效能进行评价与调整。

无论是定性鉴别还是定量测定，均要求待测物质色谱峰与内标物质色谱峰或特定的杂质对照色谱峰及其他色谱峰之间有较好的分离度。除另有规定外，待测物质色谱峰与相邻色谱峰之间的分离度应不小于1.5。分离度的计算公式为

$$R = 2 \times (t_{R_2} - t_{R_1})/(W_1 + W_2) \quad 或 \quad R = 2 \times (t_{R_2} - t_{R_1})/[1.70 \times (W_{1,h/2} + W_{2,h/2})]$$

式中，t_{R_2} 为相邻两色谱峰中后一峰的保留时间，t_{R_1} 为相邻两色谱峰中前一峰的保留时间，W_1、W_2、$W_{1,h/2}$、$W_{2,h/2}$ 分别为此相邻两色谱峰的峰宽及半高峰宽（图1-2-2）。

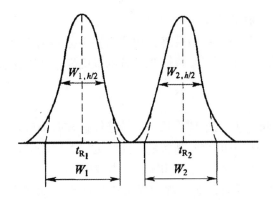

图 1-2-2 两种成分的色谱分离示意

当对测定结果有异议时，色谱柱的理论板数（n）和分离度（R）均以峰宽（W）的计算结果为准。

（三）灵敏度

灵敏度（sensitivity）用于评价色谱系统检测微量物质的能力，通常以信噪比（S/N）来表示。建立方法时，可通过测定一系列不同浓度的供试品或对照品溶液来测定信噪比。定量测定时，信噪比应不小于10；定性测定时，信噪比应不小于3。系统适用性试验中可以设置灵敏度实验溶液来评价色谱系统的检测能力。

（四）拖尾因子

拖尾因子（T）用于评价色谱峰的对称性。拖尾因子计算公式为

$$T = W_{0.05h}/2d_1$$

式中，$W_{0.05h}$ 为5%峰高处的峰宽，d_1 为峰顶在5%峰高处横坐标平行线的投影点至峰前沿与此平行线交点的距离（图1-2-3）。

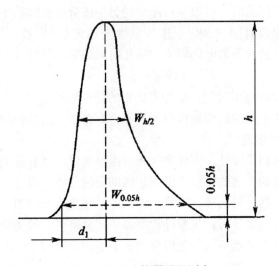

图 1-2-3 拖尾因子测定

除另有规定外，以峰高作定量参数时，T 值应为 $0.95 \sim 1.05$。

以峰面积作定量参数时，一般的峰拖尾或前伸不会影响峰面积积分，但严重拖尾会影响基线和色谱峰起止的判断和峰面积积分的准确性，此时应在品种项下对拖尾因子做出规定。

（五）重复性

重复性（repeatability）用于评价色谱系统连续进样时响应值的重复性能。采用外标法时，通常取各品种项下的对照品溶液，连续进样 5 次，除另有规定外，其峰面积测量值的相对标准偏差应不大于 2.0%；采用内标法时，通常配制相当于 80%、100% 和 120% 的对照品溶液，加入规定量的内标溶液，配成 3 种不同浓度的溶液，分别至少进样 2 次，计算平均校正因子，其相对标准偏差应不大于 2.0%。

三、测定法

（一）定性分析

1. 利用保留时间定性

保留时间（retention time，t_R）指被分离组分从进样到柱后出现该组分最大响应值的时间，即从进样到出现某组分色谱峰的顶点为止所经历的时间，常以分钟为时间单位，用于反映被分离的组分在性质上的差异。通常以在相同的色谱条件下待测成分的保留时间与对照品的保留时间是否一致作为待测成分定性的依据。

两个保留时间不同的色谱峰归属于不同化合物，但两个保留时间一致的色谱峰有时未必可归属为同一化合物，在进行未知物鉴别时应特别注意。

若改变流动相组成或更换色谱柱的种类，待测成分的保留时间仍与对照品的保留时间一致，可进一步证实待测成分与对照品为同一化合物。

当待测成分无对照品时，可以将样品中的另一成分或在样品中加入另一成分作为参比物，采用相对保留时间（RRT）作为定性（或定位）、校正因子计算含量的方法。除另有规定外，相对保留时间以未扣除死时间的非调整保留时间按下式计算：

$$RRT = t_{R_1}/t_{R_2}$$

式中，t_{R_1} 为待测成分的保留时间，t_{R_2} 为参比物的保留时间。

若需要以扣除死时间的调整保留时间计算，应在相应的品种项下予以注明。

2. 利用光谱相似度定性

化合物的全波长扫描紫外－可见光区光谱图可提供一些有价值的定性信息。待测成分的光谱与对照品的光谱的相似度可用于辅助定性分析。通过二极管阵列检测器可得到更多的信息，包括色谱信号、时间、波长的三维色谱光谱图，其既可用于辅助定性分析，还可用于峰纯度分析，与紫外检测器相比具有更大的优势。

同样应注意，两个光谱不同的色谱峰表征了不同化合物，但两个光谱相似的色谱峰未必可归属为同一化合物。

3. 利用质谱检测器定性

利用质谱检测器提供的色谱峰分子质量和结构的信息进行定性分析，可获得比仅利用保留时间或增加光谱相似性进行定性分析更多、更可靠的信息，不仅可用于已知物的定性分析，还可提供未知化合物的结构信息。

（二）定量分析

1. 内标法

精密称（量）取对照品和内标物质，分别配成溶液，各精密量取适量，混合配成校正因子测定用的对照溶液。取一定量进样，记录色谱图。测量对照品和内标物质的峰面积或峰高，按下式计算校正因子（f）：

$$f = (A_S/C_S) / (A_R/C_R)$$

式中，A_S为内标物质的峰面积或峰高，A_R为对照品的峰面积或峰高，C_S为内标物质的浓度，C_R为对照品的浓度。

再取各品种项下含有内标物质的供试品溶液，进样，记录色谱图，测量供试品中待测成分和内标物质的峰面积或峰高，按下式计算含量（C_X）：

$$C_X = f \times A_X / (A'_S/C'_S)$$

式中，A_X为供试品的峰面积或峰高，c_X为供试品的浓度，A'_S为内标物质的峰面积或峰高，C'_S为内标物质的浓度，f为内标法校正因子。采用内标法，可避免样品前处理及进样体积误差对测定结果的影响。

2. 外标法

精密称（量）取对照品和供试品，配制成溶液，分别精密称取一定量，进样，记录色谱图，测量对照品溶液和供试品溶液中待测物质的峰面积（或峰高），按下式计算含量（C_X）：

$$C_X = C_R \times A_X / A_R$$

式中，各符号意义同上式。当采用外标法测定时，以手动进样器定量环或自动进样器进样为宜。

3. 加校正因子的主成分自身对照法

测定杂质含量时，可采用加校正因子的主成分自身对照法。在建立方法时，按各品种项下的规定，精密称（量）取待测物对照品和参比物质对照品各适量，配制待测杂质校正因子的溶液，进样，记录色谱图，按下式计算待测杂质的校正因子（f）：

$$f = C_A \times A_B / (A_A \times C_B)$$

式中，C_A为待测物的浓度，A_A为待测物的峰面积或峰高，C_B为参比物质的浓度，A_B为参比物质的峰面积或峰高。

也可精密称（量）取主成分对照品和杂质对照品各适量，分别配制成不同浓度的溶液，进样，记录色谱图，绘制主成分浓度和杂质浓度对其峰面积的回归曲线，以主成分回归直线斜率与杂质回归直线斜率的比计算校正因子。

校正因子可直接载入各品种项下，用于校正杂质的实测峰面积，需要做校正计算的杂质，通常以主成分为参比，采用相对保留时间定位，其数值一并载入各品种项下。

测定杂质含量时，按各品种项下规定的杂质限度，将供试品溶液稀释成与杂质限度相当的溶液，作为对照溶液，进样，记录色谱图，必要时，调节纵坐标范围（以噪声水平可接受为限）使对照溶液的主成分色谱峰的峰高达满量程的 $10\% \sim 25\%$。除另有规定外，通常含量低于 0.5% 的杂质，峰面积测量值的相对标准偏差（RSD）应小于 10%；含量在 $0.5\% \sim 2.0\%$ 的杂质，峰面积测量值的 RSD 应小于 5%；含量大于 2% 的杂质，峰面积测量值的 RSD 应小于 2%。然后，取供试品溶液和对照溶液适量，分别进样。除另有规定外，供试品溶液的记录时间应为主成分色谱峰保留时间的 2 倍，测量供试品溶液色谱图上各杂质的峰面积，分别乘以相应的校正因子后与对照溶液主成分的峰面积比较，计算各杂质含量。

4. 不加校正因子的主成分自身对照法

测定杂质含量时，若无法获得待测杂质的校正因子，或校正因子可以忽略，也可采用不加校正因子的主成分自身对照法。同加校正因子的主成分自身对照法配制对照溶液、进样、调节纵坐标范围和计算峰面积的相对标准偏差后，取供试品溶液和对照品溶液适量，分别进样。除另有规定外，供试品溶液的记录时间应为主成分色谱峰保留时间的 2 倍，测量供试品溶液色谱图上各杂质的峰面积并与对照溶液主成分的峰面积比较，依法计算杂质含量。

5. 面积归一化法

按各品种项下的规定，配制供试品溶液，取一定量进样，记录色谱图。测量各峰的面积和色谱图上除溶剂峰以外的总色谱峰面积，计算各峰面积占总峰面积的百分比。用于杂质检查时，由于仪器响应的线性限制，峰面积归一化法一般不宜用于微量杂质的检查。如适用，也可使用其他方法如标准曲线法等，并在品种正文项下注明。

Section 5　High Performance Liquid Chromatography(HPLC)

High performance liquid chromatography (HPLC) is a method of chromatographic separation of the substance being examined, in which the mobile phase is pumped into a column packed with the stationary phase by a high-pressure pump system. The test solution injected is carried into the column by the mobile phase. All the components are separated in the column and flow through the detector. Chromatographic signals are recorded and processed by an integrator or data processing system. The flow chart of HPLC is as follows (Fig. 1 – 2 – 1):

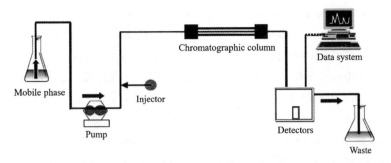

Fig. 1 −2 −1　Schematic diagram of high performance liquid chromatography

1　General Requirements for Apparatus and Chromatographic Conditions

The apparatus consists of a high-pressure pumping system, an injector, a chromatographic column, a detector and a data acquisition system. Generally, the internal diameter of columns is 3. 9 ~ 4. 6 mm and the particle size of the stationary phases is 3 ~ 10 μm. Ultra-high-performance liquid chromatography, with ultra-high-pressure resistance, small injection volume, low hold-up volume and high sensitivity detection is suitable for the column packed with small particle size(about 2 μm) of stationary phase.

1.1　Chromatographic Column

1. 1. 1　Reversed-Phase Chromatographic Column

The column packed with stationary phases using bonded non-polar groups as supports. The most widely used of supports are silica gel, polymer composite silica gel and polymers, etc. , and commonly used packing materials include octadecyl silane bonded silica gel(C_{18}) , octylsilane bonded silica gel(C_8) and phenyl bonded silica gel etc.

1. 1. 2　Normal-Phase Chromatographic Column

The column packed with stationary phases of silica gel or bonded polar group silica gel. The most widely used of stationary phases include silica gel, amino group bonded silica gel and cyano group bonded silica gel. The above three kinds of normal-phase chromatographic column also all can be used in reversed-phase chromatographic column.

1. 1. 3　Ion-Exchange Chromatographic Column

The column packed with ion exchanged stationary phases, including cation exchange chromatographic column and anion exchange chromatographic column.

1. 1. 4　Chiral Chromatographic Column

The column packed with chiral stationary phases, which can be used for the separation of chiral drugs.

The internal diameter and the length of columns, the shape of the filler, the residual surface groups of stationary phases, the particle size and distribution, the pore diameter, the surface area, the surface coverage of bonded functional groups, the density and uniform of packing, etc. , affect the performance of columns. The appropriate chromatographic column should be selected based on the characteristics of the substance being separated.

The temperature can affect separation. Unless otherwise specified in the monograph, the temperature of columns refers to room temperature (10 ～ 30 ℃) and the effect of room temperature change should be paid attention to. Columns may be heated to give higher separation efficiency. It is better that columns do not be heated above 60 ℃.

For silica gel columns with residual unblocked silico hydroxyl group, the pH value of the mobile phase is generally controlled within 2 ～ 8. For columns with residual blocked silicon hydroxyl group, or polymer composite silica gel or polymers, the mobile phase with more extensive pH value is employed. The mobile phase with pH value less than 2 or more than 8 is preferred.

1. 2 Detectors

Ultraviolet visible(UV) spectrophotometry detector, including diode array detector(DAD or PDA) , is the most commonly used detector. Fluorescence spectrophotometry detector(FD) , evaporative light scattering detector (ELSD) , charged aerosol detection (CAD) , refractive index detector(RID) , electrochemical detector(ECD) , mass spectrometry detector(MSD) may also be used.

UVD, FD and ECD are all selective detectors. The response value is related to the quantity of the substance being examined as well as its structure. ELSD, CAD and RID are general-purpose detectors, which respond to all compounds. The response value of the substance with similar structure in the ELSD is almost only related to the quantity of the substance being examined.

The response values of UVD, FD, ECD and RID are in conformity with the Lambert Beer law and linear with the amount of substance being examined within a certain range, while the relationship between the response value of the ELSD and the amount of the substance being examined is usually exponential. Therefore, it should be logarithmically transferred before calculation. The response value of the CAD usually has an exponential relationship with the amount of the substance to be measured, which usually needs to be calculated by logarithmic conversion or quadratic function, but it can be basically linear in a small mass range.

Different detectors have different requirements for the mobile phase. The mobile phase used in UVD complies with the requirements for solvents under Ultraviolet-visible Spectrophotometry(General Rule 0401) . When the light of short wavelength is applied for detection, the cut-off wavelength of the organic solvents should be considered and the organic solvent with chromatographic grade should be used. The mobile phase containing nonvolatile salts cannot be used for ELSD, CAD and MSD.

1. 3 Mobile Phase

In reversed-phase chromatograph system, the preferred mobile phase is methanol-water system and acetonitrile-water system. In case of using the ultraviolet end of the wavelength detection-water system is used as priority. The mobile phase containing buffer salts should be used as little as possible, if necessary, the low concentration of buffer salts may be used. When a column packed with octadecylsilane bonded silica gel is used, the concentration of the organic solvents in the mobile phase is not less than 5%. Otherwise it easily results in the decline of column efficiency and instability of the chromatographic system except for embedded polar group bonded stationary phase chromatographic column, etc.

Two or more than two organic solvents such as dichloromethane and n-hexane, etc., are commonly used as the mobile for normal phase chromatographic system.

The elution mode of injecting mobile phase into liquid chromatograph can be divided into two types: one is isometric elution and the other is gradient elution. When gradient elution is used, the gradient elution procedure is usually specified under the variety in the form of a table. It includes the running time and the composition ratio of the mobile phase at different times.

1.4 Chromatographic Parameter Adjustment

The type of the stationary phase, the mode of detector and the composition of the mobile phase specified in the monograph should not be changed, other items, including internal diameter and length of column, particle size of the stationary phase, flow rate and ratio of components in the mobile phase, temperature of column, injection volume and the sensitivity of detector, can be changed appropriately to meet the requirements of the system suitability test. When the ratio of components in mobile phase is adjusted, if the percentage of X component with small proportion is not more than 33%, the range of $0.7X \sim 1.3X$ is valid; if the percentage of component X is more than 33%, the range of $0.9X \sim 1.1X$ is valid.

The small particle size(about 2 μm) of the stationary phase used should be compatible with the properties of the pumping system injection volume, volume of the detection pool and hold-up volume of the system and the chromatographic conditions should be adjusted correspondingly if necessary.

The allowable adjustment range of chromatographic parameters is shown in Tab. 1 −2 −3.

Tab. 1 −2 −3 Allowable adjustment range of chromatographic column,
filler particle size and corresponding parameters

Parameter variable	Parameter adjustment
Stationary phase	The physical and chemical properties of the stationary phase must not be changed, such as filler material, surface modification and bonding phase, and the change from full porous filler to surface porous filler is allowed on the premise of meeting the above conditions

Tab. 1 – 2 – 3(Continued)

Parameter variable	Parameter adjustment
Filler particle size(dp), column length(L)	After changing the size and length of the chromatographic column, L/dp value(or N value) should be within the range of -25% and 50% of the original value
Velocity of flow	The flow rate can be adjusted within the range of $\pm 50\%$ according to the system pressure and retention time in actual use
Injection volume	Injection volume can be adjusted according to the demand of sensitivity. Even if the size of the chromatographic column is not adjusted, the injection volume can be adjusted to meet the requirements of system applicability
Gradient elution procedure (isometric elution is not applicable)	Keep the elution volume multiple of different chromatographic columns the same, so as to ensure the same gradient change, and the volume differences of different instrument systems need to be considered
Isometric elution mobile phase ratio(gradient elution is not applicable)	The minimum proportion of mobile phase components can be adjusted within the range of relative value $\pm 30\%$ or absolute value $\pm 2\%$ (choose the maximum between the two); the proportion of minimum proportion mobile phase components should be less than($100/n$)%, and n is the number of components in the mobile phase
Mobile phase buffer salt concentration	Can be adjusted in the range of $\pm 10\%$
Column temperature	When the temperature is specified, it can be adjusted in the range of ± 10 ℃
pH value	Unless otherwise specified, the pH value of the aqueous phase in the mobile phase can be adjusted within the range of ± 0.2 pH
Detection wavelength	No change allowed

The adjustment range of injection volume, flow rate and gradient elution procedure in Tab. 1 – 2 – 3 can be calculated by relevant software, and fine-tuned according to the separation of chromatographic peaks.

The possible effects of chromatographic parameter adjustment on separation and detection should be evaluated. If the adjustment goes beyond the range specified in Tab. 1 – 2 – 3, the method of adjustment should be verified accordingly. After adjustment, the applicability of the system should meet the requirements, and the order of chromatographic peaks remains unchanged. If the injection volume is reduced, the repeatability of detection limit and peak area should be ensured, and if the injection volume is increased, the degree of separation and linear relationship should still meet the requirements.

For gradient elution, the adjustment of gradient elution chromatographic parameters should be more cautious than that of isometric elution, because this adjustment may change the position of some peaks, cause peak recognition errors, or merge with other peaks.

No matter whether the adjusted method is verified or not, when there is an objection to the determination results after adjusting the chromatographic conditions, the determination results of the chromatographic conditions specified under the variety shall prevail.

Under the variety item, it is generally not suitable to specify or recommend the brand of the chromatographic column, but the type of filler(fixed phase) of the chromatographic column (such as bonding phase, whether modified, capped, etc.) , particle size, pore diameter, column length or inner diameter of the column can be specified; when the durability test proves that a specific brand of chromatographic column must be used to meet the separation requirements, it can be indicated under the text of the variety.

2　The System Suitability Test

The suitability test of the chromatographic system generally includes five parameters, which are resolution, the number of theoretical plates, sensitivity, repeatability and tailing factor.

Carry out the system suitability test in accordance with the requirements specified in the monograph, using specified reference solution or system suitability test solution under the specified chromatographic conditions, which could be adjusted to comply with the requirements if necessary.

2. 1　Number of Theoretical Plates of the Column

Number of theoretical plates of the column (n) is used to evaluate the separation performance of columns. Due to different chromatographic behaviors of different substances on the same column, using the number of theoretical plates as the parameter to evaluate the column performance, the substance being examined should be stated. Number of theoretical plates usually refers to that of the substance being examined or the internal standard.

Inject the test solution or the internal standard solution specified in the monograph into the column under the prescribe chromatographic conditions. Record the chromatogram and measure the retention time t_R and width(W) or width at half-height($W_{h/2}$) of the principle peak obtained with the test solution or the internal standard solution. Calculate number of theoretical plates of the column, using the following equation:

$$n = 16(t_R/W)^2 \text{ or } n = 5.54(t_R/W_{h/2})^2$$

The values of t_R, W and $W_{h/2}$ can be expressed in minutes or in length(same as below) , but must be expressed in the same units.

2. 2　Resolution

Resolution(R) is used to evaluate the resolution between the substance being examined and the substance being separated and it is a key parameter for evaluating the separation performance of chromatographic system. The separation performance can be evaluated and adjusted by the resolution between the substance being examined and known impurities, or by the resolution between the substance being examined and a certain index component(such as the internal standard or other substance being separated with difficultly) , or by the resolution between the substance being examined and a certain degraded product obtained with the degradation of the substance being examined or the reference substance using an appropriate method.

No matter in qualitative or quantitative determination, good resolution between peaks of the substance being examined and the internal standard or specified impurities or other substances should be achieved. Unless otherwise specified the resolution between the peak of the substance being examined and the adjacent peaks is more than 1.5. Calculate the resolution using the following equation:

$$R = 2 \times (t_{R_2} - t_{R_1}) / (W_1 + W_2) \text{ or } R = 2 \times (t_{R_2}/t_{R_1}) / [1.70 \times (W_{1,h/2} + W_{2,h/2})]$$

where t_{R_2} is the retention time of the latter of the two adjacent peaks; t_{R_1} is the retention time of the former of the two adjacent peaks; W_1, W_2, $W_{1,h/2}$, $W_{2,h/2}$ are the peak width and peak width at half height of the two adjacent peaks separately(Fig. 1 -2 -2) .

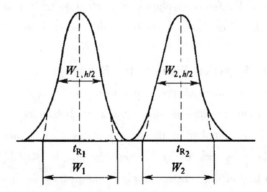

Fig. 1 -2 -2   Schematic diagram of chromatographic separation of two components

Number of theoretical plates of the column(n) and resolution(R) are calculated as peak width(W) if the determination result is disputed.

2.3   Sensitivity

Sensitivity is used to evaluate the capability of the chromatographic system for determining minute substances, usually expressed in signal-to-noise ratio(S/N) , which is obtained by determining the test solution or the reference solution with a series of different concentrations. For quantitative determination, signal-to-noise ratio is not less than 10; for qualitative determination, signal-to-noise ratio is not less than 3. The sensitivity test solution is used for evaluating the detection capability of the chromatographic system.

2.4 Tailing Factor

Tailing factor(T) is used to evaluate the symmetry of chromatographic peaks. Calculate the tailing factor using the following equation:

$$T = W_{0.05h}/2d_1$$

where $W_{0.05h}$ is the peak width at 5% of the peak height, d_1 is the distance between the perpendicular dropped from the peak maximum and the leading edge of the peak at 5% of the peak height(Fig. 1 – 2 – 3).

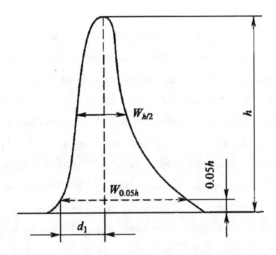

Fig. 1 – 2 – 3   Determination of tailing factor

Unless otherwise specified, the T value should be within $0.95 \sim 1.05$ by using peak height as the quantitative parameter.

Using peak area as the quantitative parameter, general peak tailing or fronting does not affect the integration of peak area. But serious peak tailing will affect the judgment of baseline and the front and the end of peak as well as the accuracy of the integration of peak area. Thus tailing factor should be stated in the monograph.

2.5 Repeatability

Repeatability is used to evaluate repeatability of the response value of chromatographic system for consecutive injections. Using the external standard method, inject the reference solution described in the monograph for 5 times consecutively, unless otherwise specified, the relative standard deviation of peak area measurement is not more than 2.0%. Using internal standard method, prepare a series of reference solutions equivalent to 80%, 100% and 120% of the concentration of the substance being examined, add specified volume of the internal standard solution separately to produce solutions with three different concentrations, inject each solution at least twice, calculate the average correction factor, and corresponding relative standard deviation is not more than 2.0%.

3 Procedure

3.1 Qualitative Analysis

3.1.1 The Qualitative Retention Time

The qualitative retention time (t_R) is defined as the time from the injection of the separated component to the maximum response value of the component after the column, that is, the time from the injection to the peak of the chromatographic peak of a certain component, which is often in minute as the time unit, which is used to reflect the differences in the properties of the separated components. The qualitative basis of the components to be tested is usually based on whether the retention time of the components to be tested is consistent with that of the reference substance under the same chromatographic conditions.

Under the same chromatographic conditions, there should be no significant difference between the retention time of the tested components and that of the control substance, and the two chromatographic peaks with different retention time should belong to different compounds. However, the two chromatographic peaks with the same retention time may not be classified as the same compound, so special attention should be paid to the identification of unknown substances.

If the composition of the mobile phase is changed or the type of the chromatographic column is changed, the retention time of the components to be tested is still the same as that of the reference substance, which can further confirm that the components to be tested are the same compound as the reference substance.

When the component to be tested (retention time t_{R_1}) has no reference substance, another component in the sample or another component can be added to the sample as a reference (retention time t_{R_2}), and the relative retention time (RRT) can be used as a qualitative (or positioning) and correction factor to calculate the content. Under the variety item, unless otherwise provided, the relative retention time shall be calculated according to the following formula based on the non-adjusted retention time without deducting the dead time:

$$RRT = t_{R_1} / t_{R_2}$$

If it is necessary to calculate the adjusted retention time after deducting the dead time, it should be indicated under the corresponding variety.

3.1.2 Qualitative Analysis by Spectral Similarity

The full-wavelength scanning UV-vis spectra of the compounds provide some valuable qualitative information. The similarity between the spectrum of the components to be measured and that of the reference substance can be used to assist qualitative analysis. The DAD can get more information, including the three-dimensional chromatogram of chromatographic signal, time and wavelength, which can be used to assist qualitative analysis, qualitative results and peak purity analysis. Compared with UVD, it has more advantages.

It should also be noted that two chromatographic peaks with different spectra represent different compounds, but two chromatographic peaks with similar spectra may not be classified as the same compound.

3. 1. 3　Using the MSD to Qualitatively Analyze

Using the MSD to qualitatively analyze the molecular weight and structure of the chromatographic peak provided by the MSD, more and more reliable information can be obtained than only using retention time or increasing spectral similarity for qualitative analysis. It can not only be used for the qualitative analysis of known substances, but also provide structural information of unknown compounds.

3. 2　Qualitative Analysis

3. 2. 1　Internal Standard Method

Prepare solutions containing an accurately weighed quantity of the reference substance and the internal standard respective as specified in the monograph. Measure an accurately volume of each solution mix well to produce the reference solution used for determination of the correction factor. Inject a certain volume of solution into the equipment and record the chromatogram.

Measure the peak area or the peak height of the reference substance and that of the internal standard, calculate the correction factor(f), using the following equation:

$$f = (A_S/C_S)/(A_R/C_R)$$

where As is the peak area or peak height of the internal standard, A_R is the peak area or peak height of the reference substance, C_s is the concentration of the internal standard, C_R is the concentration of the reference solution.

Inject the test solution containing the internal standard as described in the monograph and record the chromatogram.

Measure the peak area or the peak height of the substance being examined and that of the internal standard. Calculate the content(C_X), using the following equation:

$$C_X = f \times (A'_S/C'_S)$$

where A_X is the peak area or peak height of the substance being examined, C_X is the concentration of the solution of the substance being examined, $A's$ is the peak area or the peak height of the internal standard, $C's$ is the concentration of the internal standard solution, f is the correction factor.

Using the internal standard method, the effects on determination result due to injection volume errors can be avoid.

3. 2. 2　External Standard Method

Prepare solutions containing an accurately weighed quantity of the reference substance and the substance being examined respectively. Inject a certain volume of each solution and record the chromatograms.

Measure the peak area or peak height of the substance being examined in the reference solution and the test solution separately. Calculate the content (C_X), using the following equation:

$$C_X = C_R \times A_X/A_R$$

where each symbol has the same meaning as mentioned above.

As the microsyringe is not easy to control the injection volume precisely, if using external standard method, the manual fixed-loop or automatic sampler may be used.

3.2.3 Corrected Peak Areas of Impurities Compared with That Produced by the Main Peak of the Substance Being Examined

This method is used for determination of contents impurities. In the establishment of a method, prepare solutions containing an accurately weighed quantity of the reference substances of impurities and the reference component as specified in the monograph, mix well to produce the solution for determination of the correction factor. Inject a volume into the column and record the chromatogram. Calculate the correction factor(f) of impurities being examined, using the following equation:

$$f = C_A \times A_B/(C_B \times A_A)$$

where C_A is the concentration of the solution of impurities being examined, A_A is the peak area or peak height of impurities being examined, C_B is the concentration of the reference component solution, A_B is the peak area or peak height of the reference component.

Also prepare solutions containing an accurately weighed quantity of the main component chemical reference substance(CRS) and impurity CRS with different concentrations. Inject a volume and record the chromatogram, plot regression curves of the concentration of the main component and impurities to corresponding peak areas. Calculate the correction factor, using the ratio of regression line slope of the main component to that of impurities.

The correction factor can be directly stated in the monograph and it is used for correction of the measured peak areas of impurities. The value of impurity to be corrected should be stated in the monograph, using the main component as the reference component and the relative retention time as the location.

To determine the content of impurity, dilute the test solution to equivalent concentration of impurity limit solution, in accordance with the impurity limit indicated in the monograph, use as the reference solution. Inject a volume and record the chromatogram. If necessary, adjust the ordinate range (limited by the noise level that can be accepted) until the peak height of the main component obtained in the reference solution is about $10\% \sim 25\%$ of the full scale. Unless otherwise specified, for the impurity with content less than 0.5%, relative standard deviation(RSD) of the peak area should be less than 10%; for the impurity with content within $0.5\% \sim 2.0\%$, RSD of the peak area should be less than 5%; for the impurity with content more than 2%, RSD of the peak area should be less than 2%. Inject a volume of the test solution and the reference solution into the column separately, unless otherwise specified, the record time of the test solution is twice the retention time of the principle peak. Measure the peak areas of all impurities on the chromatogram obtained with the test solution, multiply by the corresponding correction factor separately, with respect to the peak area of the main component obtained with the reference solution, calculate the content of impurities.

3.2.4 Peak Areas of Impurities Compared with That Produced by the Main Peak of the Substance Being Examined(Self-control Method)

If correction factor of the impurities being examined is not achieved or is disregarded, this method is used to determine the content of impurities. Prepare the reference solution as indicated in above Method 3.2.3. Adjust the ordinate range and calculate RSD of peak area. Inject separately an appropriate volume of the test solution and the reference solution into the column, unless otherwise specified, the record time of the test solution is twice the retention time of the peak of the main component. Measure the peak areas of all impurities obtained in the test solution with respect to the peak area of the main component obtained in the reference solution calculate the content of impurities.

3.2.5 Peak Area Normalization Method

Prepare the test solution as specified in the monograph. Inject a certain volume into the column and record the chromatogram. Measure the peak area of each peak and all peaks other than solvent peak. Calculate the percentage of each peak area in the total area of all peaks. Due to linear limit of apparatus response, the peak area normalization method is not suitable for determination of minute impurity.

If applicable, other methods such as standard curve method can also be used and marked under the text of the variety.

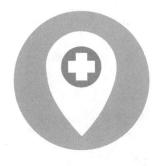

下编 ｜ 药物分析实验

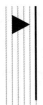

实验一 容量仪器的校正

一、目的要求

（1）了解容量仪器校正的意义。
（2）掌握容量仪器校正的方法。
（3）复习分析天平的使用方法。

二、实验原理

定量分析中应用的容量仪器，都需要很准确的容积，否则在使用时就会影响分析结果的准确性，故必须事先进行校正。

测量体积的基本单位是毫升（mL），即真空中 1 g 纯水在 4 ℃（水在 4 ℃时密度最大）时所占的体积，但 4 ℃并不是我们适宜的工作条件，故一般以 20 ℃作为标准。水的体积在 4 ℃以上时随温度上升而膨胀（玻璃容器的体积也随温度变化而变化，但玻璃膨胀系数很小，通常可以忽略不计）。在空气中称重时，因空气的浮力，重量也会减少。因此，对这些因素皆应加以校正。可以从表 2－1－1 查出相应温度时的水在空气中的质量，通过计算便可得到较准确的校正结果。

根据 20 ℃时容量为 1 L 的玻璃容器在不同温度时所盛水的质量，可计算量器的校正值。

表 2－1－1 不同温度下 1 L 水在空气中的质量

温度/℃	1 L 水在空气中的质量/g	温度/℃	1 L 水在空气中的质量/g
10	998.39	23	996.60
11	998.32	24	996.38
12	998.23	25	996.17
13	998.14	26	995.93
14	998.04	27	995.69
15	997.93	28	995.44
16	997.80	29	995.18

续表 2 - 1 - 1

温度/℃	1 L 水在空气中的质量/g	温度/℃	1 L 水在空气中的质量/g
17	997.66	30	994.91
18	997.51	31	994.64
19	997.35	32	994.34
20	997.18	33	994.06
21	997.00	34	994.75
22	996.80	35	993.45

三、实验仪器与试剂

蒸馏水、50 mL 滴定管、50 mL 量瓶、10 mL 移液管、250 mL 具塞锥形瓶、分析天平、温度计。

四、实验步骤

(一) 滴定管的校正

将蒸馏水预先放在天平室内，使其达到室温，测量其温度，然后将水装入已洗净的滴定管中，调节水至零刻度处，再按一定的滴定速度（每秒 3～4 滴）放出一定体积的水到已称量的具塞锥形瓶中，再称量，两次质量差是水的质量。根据表 2 - 1 - 1 中实验温度时水的密度，即可算出水的真实体积。按国家计量局规定，常量滴定管分 5 段进行校正。现以校正 50 mL 滴定管为例，举一试验数据列于表 2 - 1 - 2。

表 2 - 1 - 2　50 mL 滴定管的校正（温度为 18 ℃，水的密度为 0.997 51 g/mL）

滴定管读取容积/mL	瓶 + 水的质量/g	空瓶的质量/g	水的质量/g	真实容积/mL	校正值/mL
0.00～10.00	44.74	34.80	9.94	9.97	-0.03
0.00～20.00	64.64	44.74	19.90	19.95	-0.05
0.00～30.00	94.49	64.64	29.85	29.92	-0.08
0.00～40.00	74.77	34.90	39.87	39.97	-0.03
0.00～50.00	84.73	34.88	49.98	49.98	-0.02

(二) 量瓶的校正

将待校正的量瓶洗净并干燥，取烧杯并加入一定量蒸馏水，将量瓶及蒸馏水同时放于天平室中一段时间，使其温度与室温一致，记下蒸馏水的温度。先将空量瓶连同瓶塞称重（可用千分之一天平称准至四位有效数字即可），然后加蒸馏水至刻度，注意刻度之上不可留有水珠，否则应用干燥滤纸擦干，塞上瓶塞，再称重，减去空瓶质量即得量瓶中水的质量，用表2-1-1中实验温度时水的密度求得水的真实体积。

（三）移液管的校正

取内壁已洗净的移液管，按照移液管的使用方法，吸取蒸馏水至刻度线上，调节水面至刻度，然后将蒸馏水放入已称重的锥形瓶中，称重，记下蒸馏水的温度，从表2-1-1查出水的密度，以此密度除放出水的质量，即得移液管的真实体积。

［附］容量仪器的允许误差范围

国家计量局规定了常用滴定分析仪器的允差（20 ℃）。滴定管、量瓶、移液管的允差见表2-1-3至表2-1-5。

表2-1-3　滴定管的允差

单位：mL

规格		5	10	25	50	100
允差	一等	±0.01	±0.02	±0.03	±0.05	±0.10
	二等	±0.03	±0.04	±0.06	±0.10	±0.20

表2-1-4　量瓶的允差

单位：mL

规格		10	25	50	100	200	250	500	1 000	2 000
允差	一等	±0.02	±0.03	±0.05	±0.10	±0.10	±0.10	±0.15	±0.30	±0.50
	二等	±0.04	±0.06	±0.10	±0.20	±0.20	±0.20	±0.30	±0.60	±1.01

表2-1-5　移液管的允差

单位：mL

规格		1	2	5	10	15	20	25	40	50	100
允差	一等	±0.006	±0.006	±0.01	±0.02	±0.03	±0.04	±0.05	±0.05	±0.05	±0.08
	二等	±0.015	±0.015	±0.02	±0.04	±0.06	±0.10	±0.12	±0.12	±0.12	±0.16

五、注意事项

（1）所用蒸馏水至少应在天平室内放置1 h以上。

（2）待校正的仪器，应仔细洗涤至内壁完全不挂水珠（常用洗液洗涤）。

（3）校正时所用的锥形瓶，必须干净，瓶外须干燥。

（4）一般每个仪器应校正2次，即做平行试验2次。

（5）由滴定管放出水时，勿将水滴在磨口上。

（6）滴定管、移液管的操作一定要正确。

六、思考题

（1）为什么要进行容量仪器的校正？

（2）在开始放水前，若滴定管和移液管尖端或外壁挂有水珠，应怎样处理？

（3）分段校准滴定管时，为何每次要从 0.00 mL 开始？

（4）称量时应将天平箱内干燥剂取出，为什么？

（5）校正容量瓶、移液管、滴定管时，这些玻璃仪器是否均需要预先干燥？为什么？

Experiment 1 The Calibration of Volumetric Instruments

1 Purposes

(1) To understand the significance of the calibration of volumetric instruments.

(2) To learn about the methods of the calibration of volumetric instruments.

(3) To review the operation method of the analytical balance.

2 Principles

The volumetric instruments used in quantitative analysis must have a very accurate volume. Otherwise, the accuracy of the analysis results will be affected when they are used without calibration in advance.

The basic unit of volume measurement is milliliter(mL)—the volume of 1 g pure water in vacuum at 4 ℃(the water reach the highest density at 4 ℃), but this temperature is not our suitable working conditions, so we generally take 20 ℃ as the standard. When the temperature of water is above 4 ℃, its volume expands with the increase of temperature. (The volume of a glass container also varies with temperature, but the expansion coefficient of the glass is so small that it is usually negligible.) Weighing in the air, the weight of the liquid will also decrease because of the buoyancy of the air. Therefore, all these factors should be corrected. We can find out the weight of water in the air at the corresponding temperature from the water density table(Tab. 2 – 1 – 1), and get more accurate corrected results by calculation. According to the weight of water at different temperatures, which contained in a glass container with a capacity of 1 L at 20 ℃ (Tab. 2 – 1 – 1), we can calculate the corrected volume of the volumetric instrument.

Tab. 2 – 1 – 1 The weight of 1 L water at different temperatures

Temperature/℃	The weight of 1 L water in the air/g	Temperature/℃	The weight of 1 L water in the air/g
10	998. 39	23	996. 60
11	998. 32	24	996. 38
12	998. 23	25	996. 17
13	998. 14	26	995. 93
14	998. 04	27	995. 69
15	997. 93	28	995. 44

Tab. 2 – 1 – 1(Continued)

Temperature/℃	The weight of 1 L water in the air/g	Temperature/℃	The weight of 1 L water in the air/g
16	997. 80	29	995. 18
17	997. 66	30	994. 91
18	997. 51	31	994. 64
19	997. 35	32	994. 34
20	997. 18	33	994. 06
21	997. 00	34	994. 75
22	996. 80	35	993. 45

3　Instruments and Reagents

Distilled water, 50 mL burette, 50 mL volumetric flask, 10 mL pipette, 250 mL stoppered conical flask, electronic balance, thermometer.

4　Experimental Procedures

4.1　The Calibration of the Burette

The distilled water will be put in the balance room to make it reach the room temperature before measure its temperature. Then put the water into the washed burette, adjust the horizontal plane to zero graduation line, and then release a certain volume of water into the weighed stoppered conical flask at a certain titration rate(3 ~ 4 drops per second). Weigh again, we can get the weight of water from the difference between the two weights. According to the density of water at the experimental temperature in the Tab. 2 – 1 – 1, we can obtain the real volume of the water. According to the State Bureau of Metrology, constant burette could be corrected in five stages. Now we take 50 mL burette as an example, list the test data in Tab. 2 – 1 – 2.

Tab. 2 – 1 – 2　The calibration of the 50 mL burette(at 18 ℃, the density of water is 0. 997 51 g/mL)

Volume of burette reading/mL	Weight of bottle + water/g	Weight of empty bottle/g	Weight of water/g	Real volume/mL	Corrected volume/mL
0. 00 ~ 10. 00	44. 74	34. 80	9. 94	9. 97	– 0. 03
0. 00 ~ 20. 00	64. 64	44. 74	19. 90	19. 95	– 0. 05
0. 00 ~ 30. 00	94. 49	64. 64	29. 85	29. 92	– 0. 08
0. 00 ~ 40. 00	74. 77	34. 90	39. 87	39. 97	– 0. 03
0. 00 ~ 50. 00	84. 73	34. 88	49. 98	49. 98	– 0. 02

4.2 The Calibration of the Volumetric Flask

Wash and dry the flask to be calibrated, put a certain amount of distilled water into the flask. Put the flask and distilled water in the balance room at the same time for a while until the temperature is consistent with the air temperature and record the temperature. Firstly, weigh the empty bottle together with the stopper(1/1 000 balance can be used to weigh up adjusted to four-digit number), then add distilled water to the graduation line without any water droplet left above the graduation line. Otherwise, use dry filter paper to dry it and plug the stopper, then weigh. The weight of water in the volumetric flask can be obtained by subtracting the weight of empty bottles. The real volume of water can be calculated using the density of water at the experimental temperature in the Tab. 2 – 1 – 1.

4.3 The Calibration of the Pipette

Take the pipette with washed inner wall, according to the pipette use method, draw distilled water until higher than the calibration line and adjust the water surface to the line. Put the distilled water into a weighed conical flask, weigh, and record the temperature of distilled water. Find out the density of water at this temperature in the Tab. 2 – 1 – 1, and the real volume of the pipette can be obtained with the weight of the water divided by the density.

Attachment: tolerance error range of volumetric instruments.

The State Bureau of Metrology provides the allowable error of commonly used volumetric instruments(20 ℃). The following(Tab. 2 – 1 – 3 to Tab. 2 – 1 – 5) is the allowable error of the burette, volumetric flask and pipette.

Tab. 2 – 1 – 3   The allowable error of the burette(mL)

Specification		5	10	25	50	100
Allowable error	First class	±0.01	±0.02	±0.03	±0.05	±0.10
	Second class	±0.03	±0.04	±0.06	±0.10	±0.20

Tab. 2 – 1 – 4   The allowable error of the volumetric flask(mL)

Specification		10	25	50	100	200	250	500	1000	2000
Allowable error	First class	±0.02	±0.03	±0.05	±0.10	±0.10	±0.10	±0.15	±0.30	±0.50
	Second class	±0.04	±0.06	±0.10	±0.20	±0.20	±0.20	±0.30	±0.60	±1.01

Tab. 2 −1 −5　The allowable error of the pipette(mL)

Specification		1	2	5	10	15	20	25	40	50	100
Allowable error	First class	±0. 006	±0. 006	±0. 01	±0. 02	±0. 03	±0. 04	±0. 05	±0. 05	±0. 05	±0. 08
	Second class	±0. 015	±0. 015	±0. 02	±0. 04	±0. 06	±0. 10	±0. 12	±0. 12	±0. 12	±0. 16

5　Precautions

(1) The distilled water should be placed in the balance room for 1 h at least before it is used.

(2) The instruments to be calibrate should be carefully washed until there is no water droplet hanging inside the wall(commonly using the cleaning fluid).

(3) The tapered flask used for calibration must be clean and dry outside the bottle.

(4) Each instrument should be corrected 2 times generally, that is, do parallel tests 2 times.

(5) Do not drop water on the grinding mouth when discharging water from burette.

(6) The operation of burette and pipette must be correct.

6　Questions

(1) Why do we need to calibrate the volumetric instruments?

(2) What should we do if there are water droplets on the burette and pipette tip or outer wall before launching?

(3) Why we begin at 0. 00 mL every time when we calibrate the titration pipette?

(4) Why should we remove the desiccant from the balance box when weighing?

(5) Do these glass instruments need to be dried beforehand when calibrating the burette, pipettes and volumetric flask? Why?

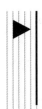

实验二 葡萄糖的分析

一、目的要求

（1）了解葡萄糖的全检过程。

（2）掌握氯化物、硫酸盐、铁盐、重金属、砷盐及炽灼残渣等一般杂质检验的基本原理、操作方法及杂质限量计算。

（3）掌握旋光法测定葡萄糖注射液含量的基本原理、操作方法及结果计算。

（4）正确使用纳氏比色管、检砷器、马弗炉及旋光仪，熟悉旋光仪的构造、工作原理及保养方法。

二、实验原理

本品为 D – （+）–吡喃葡萄糖一水合物（图2 – 2 – 1）。

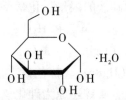

图2 – 2 – 1 葡萄糖（Glucose，$C_6H_{12}O_6 \cdot H_2O$，FW = 198.17）

葡萄糖分子结构中的 5 个碳都是手性碳原子，具有旋光性。一定条件下的旋光度是旋光性物质的特性常数，测定葡萄糖的比旋度具有初步鉴别及估测纯度的意义。

葡萄糖分子中具有醛基，可还原碱性酒石酸铜生成红色氧化亚铜沉淀。

葡萄糖分子中的官能团如羟基、亚甲基、羰基等在红外光谱中都有非常明确的特征吸收峰，可用于葡萄糖的鉴别。

（一）氯化物检查法

氯化物在硝酸酸性溶液中与硝酸银作用，生成氯化银微粒而显白色浑浊，将其与一定量的标准氯化钠溶液和硝酸银在同样的条件下用同法处理生成的氯化银浑浊程度相比较，测定供试品中氯化物的限量。化学反应式为：

$Cl^- + Ag^+ \rightarrow AgCl\downarrow$

（二）硫酸盐检查法

药物中微量硫酸盐与氯化钡在酸性溶液中反应，生成硫酸钡微粒而显白色浑浊液，将其与一定量的标准硫酸钾溶液和氯化钡在同样条件下用同法处理生成的浑浊比较，判断药物中硫酸盐的限量。化学反应式为：

$$SO_4^{2-} + Ba^{2+} \rightarrow BaSO_4 \downarrow$$

（三）铁盐检查法

三价铁盐在硝酸酸性溶液中与硫氰酸盐生成红色可溶性的硫氰酸铁络合离子，将其与一定量标准铁溶液用同法处理后进行比色。加硝酸 3 滴，煮沸 5 min，可使 Fe^{2+} 氧化成 Fe^{3+}。化学反应式为：

$$Fe^{3+} + 6SCN^- \rightarrow [Fe(SCN)_6]^{3-}$$

（四）重金属检查法

重金属是指在弱酸性（pH 3.0 ～ 3.5）溶液中，能与硫代乙酰胺或硫化钠作用生成硫化物的金属杂质。在药品生产中遇到铅的机会较多，铅又易积蓄中毒，故检查时以铅为代表。同上法，硫代乙酰胺分别和样品、对照品生成铅的硫化物的均匀沉淀，再比较判断样品中的重金属限量。化学反应式为：

$$CH_3CSNH_2 + H_2O \rightarrow CH_3CONH_2 + H_2S \uparrow$$

$$Pb^{2+} + H_2S \rightarrow PbS \downarrow + 2H^+$$

（五）砷盐检查法

利用金属锌与酸作用产生新生态的氢，将其与药物中微量砷盐作用生成具挥发性的砷化氢，砷化氢遇溴化汞试纸，产生黄色至棕色的砷斑，将其与一定量标准砷溶液所生成的砷斑比较，判断药物中砷盐的限量。化学反应式为：

$$AsO_3^{3-} + 3Zn + 9H^+ \rightarrow AsH_3 \uparrow + 3Zn^{2+} + 3H_2O$$

$$AsH_3 + 2HgBr_2 \rightarrow 2HBr + AsH(HgBr)_2（黄色）$$

$$AsH_3 + 3HgBr_2 \rightarrow 3HBr + As(HgBr)_3（棕色）$$

五价砷在酸性溶液中也能被金属锌还原为砷化氢，但生成砷化氢的速度较三价砷慢，故在反应液中加入碘化钾及酸性氯化亚锡将五价砷还原为三价砷酸根，碘化钾被氧化生成的碘又可被氯化亚锡还原为碘离子。溶液中的碘离子，与反应中产生的锌离子可形成配合物，使生成砷化氢的反应不断进行。化学反应式为：

$$AsO_4^{3-} + 2I^- + 2H^+ \rightarrow AsO_3^{3-} + I_2 + H_2O;$$

$$AsO_4^{3-} + Sn^{2+} + 2H^+ \rightarrow AsO_3^{3-} + Sn^{4+} + H_2O$$

$$I_2 + Sn^{2+} \rightarrow 2I^- + Sn^{4+};$$

$$4I^- + Zn^{2+} \rightarrow ZnI_4^{2-}$$

（六）炽灼残渣检查法

有机药物经炽灼炭化，再加硫酸湿润、低温加热至硫酸蒸气除尽，于高温（700 ～ 800 ℃）炽灼至完全灰化，使有机质破坏分解变为挥发性物质逸出，残留的非挥发性无机杂质（多为金属的氧化物或无机盐类）成为硫酸盐，称为炽灼残渣。

若炽灼残渣需要留作重金属检查，控制炽灼温度在 500 ～ 600 ℃，否则，将使重金属检查结果偏低。

（七）旋光法测定葡萄糖的基本原理

葡萄糖分子结构中 5 个碳都是手性碳原子，具有旋光性。当平面偏振光通过该具有光学活性的化合物溶液时，能引起旋光现象，使偏振光的平面向左或向右旋转。此种旋转在一定条件下，有一定的度数，称为旋光度，它是旋光性物质的特性常数，测定葡萄糖的比旋度具有初步鉴别及估测纯度的意义。

旋光度（α）与溶液的浓度（c）和偏振光透过溶液的厚度（L）成正比。当偏振光通过厚 1 dm 且每 1 mL 中含有旋光性物质 1 g 的溶液时，使用光线波长为钠光 D 线（589.3 nm）测量。测定温度为 t ℃时，测得的旋光度称为该物质的比旋度，以 $[\alpha]_D^t$ 表示。

葡萄糖的比旋度为 +52.750°，因此测定葡萄糖溶液的旋光度可以求得其含量。

三、实验仪器与试剂

（一）仪器
100 mL 量瓶、旋光仪、纳氏比色管、试砷瓶、扁形称量瓶、干燥箱、坩埚、马弗炉、干燥器、天平。

（二）试剂
乙醇、氨试液、碱性酒石酸铜试液、酚酞指示液、氢氧化钠滴定液、比色用氯化钴溶液、比色用重铬酸钾溶液、比色用硫酸铜溶液、碘试液、磺基水杨酸溶液、稀硝酸、标准氯化钠溶液、硝酸银试液、盐酸、标准硫酸钾溶液、氯化钡溶液、硫氰酸铵溶液、标准铁溶液、标准铅溶液、醋酸盐缓冲液、硫代乙酰胺试液、稀硫酸、溴化钾溴试液、碘化钾试液、酸性氯化锡试液、标准砷溶液、葡萄糖、葡萄糖注射液、可溶性淀粉。

四、实验步骤

（一）性状
葡萄糖为无色结晶，或白色结晶性或颗粒性粉末，无臭，味甜。在水中易溶，乙醇中微溶。

取葡萄糖约 10 g，精密称定，置 100 mL 量瓶中，加水适量与氨试液 0.2 mL，溶解后，用水稀释至刻度，摇匀，放置 10 min，在 25 ℃时测定比旋度，应为 +52.6°～+53.2°。

（二）鉴别
（1）取葡萄糖约 0.2 g，加水 5 mL 溶解后，缓缓滴入温热的碱性酒石酸铜试液中，即生成氧化亚铜红色沉淀。

（2）葡萄糖的红外光吸收图谱应与图 2-2-2 一致。

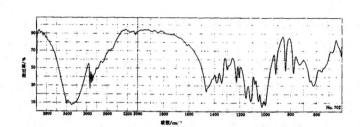

图 2-2-2 葡萄糖的红外光谱对照图谱

（三）检查

1. 酸度

取葡萄糖 2.0 g，加新沸过的冷蒸馏水 20 mL 溶解后，加酚酞指示液 3 滴与氢氧化钠滴定液（0.02 mol/L）0.20 mL，应显粉红色。

2. 溶液的澄清度与颜色

取葡萄糖 5 g，置 25 mL 纳氏比色管中，加热水溶解后，放冷，用水稀释至 10 mL，溶液应澄清无色；若显浑浊，与 1 号浊度标准液比较，不得更浓；若显色，与对照液（取比色用氯化钴溶液 3 mL，比色用重铬酸钾溶液 3 mL 与比色用硫酸铜溶液 6 mL，加水稀释成 50 mL）1.0 mL 加水稀释至 10 mL 比较，颜色不得更深。

3. 乙醇溶液的澄清度

取葡萄糖 1.0 g，加乙醇 20 mL，置水浴上加热回流约 10 min，溶液应澄清。

4. 亚硫酸盐与可溶性淀粉

取葡萄糖 1.0 g，加水 10 mL 溶解后，加碘试液 1 滴，应立即显黄色。

5. 干燥失重

取葡萄糖 1~2 g，置于供试品同样条件下干燥至恒重的扁形称量瓶中，使供试品平铺于瓶底，厚度不超过 5 mm，加盖，精密称定。将称量瓶放入洁净的培养皿中，瓶盖半开或置瓶旁，放入（105±2）℃干燥箱中干燥。取出后迅速盖好瓶盖，置干燥器内放冷至室温，迅速精密称重（放置时间与称重顺序与空称量瓶一致）。再于（105±2）℃干燥箱中干燥至恒重，即得。减失重量为 7.5%~9.5%〔《中国药典》（2020 年版）通则 0831〕。

6. 蛋白质

取葡萄糖 1.0 g，加水 10 mL 溶解后，加磺基水杨酸溶液（1→5）3 mL，不得发生沉淀。

7. 氯化物

取葡萄糖 0.6 g，加水溶解使成 25 mL（溶液若显碱性，可滴加硝酸使其成中性），再加稀硝酸 10 mL，溶液若不澄清，应滤过，置 50 mL 纳氏比色管中，加水至 40 mL，摇匀，得供试液。另取标准氯化钠溶液 6.0 mL，置 50 mL 纳氏比色管中，加水至 40 mL，摇匀，得对照溶液。于对照溶液与供试溶液中，分别加入硝酸银试液 1.0 mL，加水稀释至 50 mL，摇匀，在暗处放置 5 min，同置黑色背景上，从比色管上方向下观察、比较，供试液颜色不得比对照溶液更浓（0.01%）。

8. 硫酸盐

取葡萄糖 2.0 g，加水溶解使成 40 mL（溶液若显碱性，可滴加盐酸使其成中性），溶液若不澄清，应滤过，置 50 mL 纳氏比色管中，加稀盐酸 2 mL，摇匀，得供试溶液。另取标准硫酸钾溶液 2.0 mL，置 50 mL 纳氏比色管中，加水至 40 mL，加稀盐酸 2 mL，摇匀，得标准溶液。于对照溶液与供试溶液中，分别加入 25% 氯化钡溶液 5 mL，用水稀释至 50 mL，充分摇匀，在暗处放置 10 min，同置黑色背景上，从比色管上方向下观察、比较，供试液颜色不得比对照溶液更浓（0.01%）。

9. 铁盐

取葡萄糖 2.0 g，加 20 mL 水溶解后，加硝酸 3 滴，缓缓煮沸 5 min，放冷，加水稀释成 45 mL，加硫氰酸铵溶液 3 mL，摇匀，若显色，与标准铁溶液 2.0 mL 用同一方法制成的对照溶液比较，颜色不得更深（0.01%）。

10. 重金属

取 50 mL 纳氏比色管两支，甲管中加标准铅溶液（10 μg/mL）2 mL 与醋酸盐缓冲液（pH 3.5）2 mL 后，加水稀释至 25 mL。取葡萄糖 4.0 g，置于乙管中，加水 23 mL 溶解后，加醋酸盐缓冲液（pH 3.5）2 mL；若供试液带颜色，可在甲管中滴加少量的稀焦糖溶液或其他无干扰的有色溶液，使之与乙管一致；再在甲乙两管中分别加硫代乙酰胺试液各 2 mL，摇匀，放置 2 min，同置白纸上，自上向下透视，乙管中显出的颜色与甲管比较，颜色不得更深（含重金属不得超过万分之五）。

11. 砷盐

取葡萄糖 2.0 g 置试砷瓶中，加水 5 mL 溶解后，加稀硫酸 5 mL 与溴化钾溴试液 0.5 mL，置水浴上加热 20 min，使保持稍过量的溴存在，必要时，再补加溴化钾溴试液适量，并随时补充蒸散的水分，放冷，加盐酸 5 mL 与水适量至 28 mL，加碘化钾试液 5 mL 与酸性氯化锡试液 5 滴。在室温下放置 10 min 后，加锌粒 2 g，迅速将瓶塞塞紧（瓶塞上已置有醋酸铅棉花及溴化汞试纸的试砷管），并在 25～40 ℃ 的水浴中反应 45 min，取出溴化汞试纸，将生成的砷斑与标准砷溶液制成的砷斑比较，颜色不得更深（0.000 1%）。

标准砷斑的制备：精密量取标准砷溶液（1 μg/mL）2 mL，于另一个试砷瓶中，加盐酸 5 mL 与蒸馏水 21 mL，照上述方法操作。

12. 炽灼残渣

取葡萄糖 1.0～2.0 g，放置到已炽灼至恒重的坩埚中，精密称定，缓缓炽烧至完全炭化，放冷至室温，加硫酸 0.5～1.0 mL 使其湿润，低温加热至硫酸蒸气被除尽，于高温（700～800 ℃）炽灼至完全灰化，移置干燥器内，放冷至室温，精密称定后，再高温（700～800 ℃）炽灼至恒重，所得炽灼残渣不得超过 0.1%。

（四）含量测定

精密量取葡萄糖注射液适量（约相当于葡萄糖 10 g），置 100 mL 量瓶中，加氨试液 0.2 mL（10% 或 10% 以下规格的本品可直接取样测定），用水稀释至刻度，摇匀，静置 10 min。

取出旋光计的测定管，用供试液冲洗数次，缓缓注入供试液适量（注意勿使产生气泡），加盖密封后，置于旋光计内，缓缓旋转检偏镜检视，至视野中均匀明亮，读取刻度盘上表示的度数，即得供试液的旋光度，使偏振光向右旋转者（顺时针方向）为右旋，以"＋"符号表示，使偏振光向左旋转者（反时针方向）为左旋，以"－"符号表示，用同法读取旋光度 3 次以上，取其平均数。

按同法测定蒸馏水的读数为空白，测得的旋光度与 2.085 2 相乘，即得供试液中含有 $C_6H_{12}O_6 \cdot H_2O$ 的质量（g）。

药典规定含葡萄糖（$C_6H_{12}O_6 \cdot H_2O$）应为标示量的 95.0%～105.0%。

五、注意事项

（1）比色或比浊操作，一般均应在纳氏比色管中进行。选择比色管时，应注意样品管与标准管的体积相等，玻璃色泽一致，管上刻度均匀，高低一致，若有差别，不得超过 2 mm。

（2）样品液与对照品液的操作应遵循平行操作的原则，并应注意按操作顺序加入各种试剂。

（3）比色、比浊前应使比色管内的试剂充分混匀，然后将两管同置于黑色或白色背景上，自上而下观察。

（4）砷盐检查时，取用的样品管与标准管应力求一致，管的长短、内径一定要相同，以免生成的色斑大小不同，影响比色。锌粒加入后，应立即将试砷管盖上、塞紧，以免 AsH_3 气体逸出。

（5）炽灼残渣时，恒重操作条件如所用的干燥器、坩埚置干燥器内放置时间等，必须一致。

（6）pH 测定时，每次在更换标准缓冲液或供试液前，应用纯化水充分洗涤电极，然后将水吸尽，也可用所换的标准缓冲液或供试液洗涤。配制标准缓冲液与溶解供试品的水应是新沸过的冷蒸馏水，其 pH 应为 5.5～7.0。

（7）旋光仪接通电源后需要预热 5～20 min。每次测定前后应用溶剂做空白校正。配制溶液及测定时，均应调节温度至（20±0.5）℃（除另有规定外）。供试溶液应澄清，若显浑浊或含有混悬的小粒，应预先滤过，并弃去初滤液。旋光管装样时应注意光路中不应有气泡，使用后应立即用水洗净晾干，切勿用刷子刷，也不能用高温烘烤。

（8）标示量，即规格量、处方量，表示单位制剂内（如每片、每丸、每毫升、每瓶等）所含主药的量。

六、思考题

（1）鉴别检查在药品质量控制中的意义及一般杂质检查的主要项目是什么？

（2）比色比浊操作应遵循的原则是什么？

（3）试根据重金属的限量及标准铅的浓度计算葡萄糖重金属检查中标准铅溶液的取用量。

（4）古蔡氏检砷法〔《中国药典》（2020年版）通则0822第一法〕中所加各试剂的作用与操作注意点是什么？

（5）根据样品取用量、杂质限量及标准砷溶液的浓度，计算标准砷溶液的取用量。

（6）什么是恒重？炽灼残渣测定的成败关键是什么？

（7）药物的一般杂质检查中，为什么称取样品时采用精度为百分之一天平即可，而坩埚的称重需要用万分之一天平？

（8）古蔡氏检砷法〔《中国药典》（2020年版）通则0822第一法〕检查砷盐，能适用于所有的药物吗？为什么？

（9）葡萄糖注射液为何要检查5-羟甲基糠醛？

（10）注射液的全检过程有什么特点？

（11）葡萄糖原料旋光度法测定比旋度时，为什么要加氨试液并放置后进行测定，而10%的葡萄糖注射液测定比旋度时却不用加氨试液？

（12）推算出旋光度法测定葡萄糖含量时的计算系数2.085 2。

Experiment 2　The Analysis of the Glucose

1　Purposes

（1）To learn about the process of the whole examination of glucose.

（2）To study basic principles, operation methods and impurity limit calculation of general impurities such as chloride, sulfate, iron salt, heavy metal, arsenic salt and ignition residue.

（3）To study the principles, procedures and calculations for the assay of chiral drugs by the measurement of optical rotation.

（4）To use Nessler's colorimetric tube, arsenic detector, Muffle furnace and polarimeter correctly and familiar with the structure, working principle and maintenance methods of the polarimeter.

2　Principles

The product is D-(+)-glucopyranose monohydrate(Fig. 2 – 2 – 1).

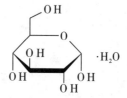

Fig. 2 – 2 – 1　Glucose($C_6H_{12}O_6 \cdot H_2O$, FW = 198. 17)

The five carbons in the structure of glucose are chiral carbon atoms with optical activity. Under certain conditions, the optical rotation is the characteristic constant of the optical substance. So, it is of great significant to determine the specific rotation of glucose in preliminary identification and estimation of purity.

The glucose molecule has aldehyde groups, which reduces copper in alkaline tartaric acid to form red cuprous oxide precipitates.

The functional groups in glucose such as hydroxyl, methylene, carbonyl, etc., have very clear characteristic absorption peaks in infrared spectrum, which can be used to identify glucose.

2. 1 Chloride

The chloride reacts with silver nitrate in nitric acid solution to form silver chloride particles which shows white turbidity. Compared with the turbidity of silver chloride produced by a certain amount of standard sodium chloride solution reacting with silver nitrate by the same method, determine the chloride limits in samples.

$$Cl^- + Ag^+ \rightarrow AgCl \downarrow$$

2. 2 Sulfate

The trace sulfate reacts with barium chloride in acidic solution results in the formation of barium sulfate particles and a white turbid solution. Compared with the turbidity produced by a certain amount of standard potassium sulfate solution reacting with barium chloride by the same method, determine the limit of sulphate content in drugs.

$$SO_4^{2-} + Ba^{2+} \rightarrow BaSO4 \downarrow$$

2. 3 Iron

Ferric salts react with thiocyanate to form red soluble iron thiocyanate complex ion in nitric acid solution. The colorimetric measurement is made by a certain amount of standard iron solution with the same treatment. Adding 3 drops of nitric acid and boiling for 5 min can make Fe^{2+} oxidize to Fe^{3+}.

$$Fe^{3+} + 6SCN^- \rightarrow [Fe(SCN)_6]^{3-}$$

2. 4 Heavy Metals

Heavy metals are impurities that can react with thioacetamide or sodium sulfide to form sulfides in weak acidic solutions(pH 3. 0 ～ 3. 5). Lead is more likely to be encountered in the production of drugs, and lead is easy to accumulate poisoning, so lead is the representative of inspection. In the same way, thioacetamide precipitates lead sulfide with the sample and standard sample respectively, and then compare and calculate the limit of heavy metals in the sample.

$$CH_3CSNH_2 + H_2O \rightarrow CH_3CONH_2 + H_2S \uparrow$$
$$Pb^{2+} + H_2S \rightarrow PbS \downarrow + 2H^+$$

2.5 As

Zn reacts with acids and nascent hydrogen is produced. Then nascent hydrogen reacts with arsonium compound and As hydride is produced. At last, As hydride reacts with the test paper of $HgBr_2$ and yellow or light brown spot of As appeared. Colors of spots of As obtained from the sample and from the standard As solution were compared to determine the As content in the sample.

$$AsO_3^{3-} + 3Zn + 9H^+ \rightarrow AsH_3 \uparrow + 3Zn^{2+} + 3H_2O$$
$$AsH_3 + 2HgBr_2 \rightarrow 2HBr + AsH(HgBr)_2 \text{ (yellow)}$$
$$AsH_3 + 3HgBr_2 \rightarrow 3HBr + As(HgBr)_3 \text{ (brown)}$$

Pentavalent As can also be reduced to hydrogen arsenide by metallic zinc in acidic solution, but the rate of formation of hydrogen arsenide is slower than that of trivalent As. Therefore, add the potassium iodide and acidic stannous chloride to the reaction solution to reduce pentavalent As to trivalent As, and the iodine produced by oxidation of potassium iodide can be reduced to iodine ion by stannous chloride. Iodine ions in the solution, and zinc ions produced in the reaction can form complex, so that the formation of hydrogen arsenide reaction continues.

$$AsO_4^{3-} + 2I^- + 2H^+ \rightarrow AsO_3^{3-} + I_2 + H_2O$$
$$AsO_4^{3-} + Sn^{2+} + 2H^+ \rightarrow AsO_3^{3-} + Sn^{4+} + H_2O$$
$$I_2 + Sn^{2+} \rightarrow 2I^- + Sn^{4+}$$
$$4I^- + Zn^{2+} \rightarrow ZnI_4^{2-}$$

2.6 Residue on Ignition

Organic medicines are charred by incandescence, then moistened by sulphuric acid and heated at low temperatures until the sulphuric acid vapor is removed. At high temperatures (700 ~ 800 ℃), they are incandescent to complete ashing, causing the destruction of organic matter to decompose into volatile substances, and the remaining non-volatile inorganic impurities (mostly metal oxides or inorganic salts) become sulphates, called residue on ignition. If the residue on ignition is kept for heavy metal test, the burning temperature should be controlled between 500 ℃ and 600 ℃. Otherwise, the result of heavy metal test will be lower.

2.7 The Basic Principle of Polarimetry for Determination of Glucose

The five carbon molecules in the glucose molecule are chiral carbon atoms with optical activity. When the planar polarized light passes through the optically active compound solution, it can cause revolving light phenomenon and make the planar plane of the polarized light rotate left or right. Under certain conditions, this rotation has a certain degree, called optical rotation, which is the characteristic constant of optical substances. The determination of specific rotation of glucose has the significance of preliminary identification and estimation of purity.

The optical rotation(α) is proportional to the concentration(C) of the solution and the thickness(L) of the polarized light through the solution. When polarized light passes through a solution 1 dm thick and contains 1 g per mL of rotatory substance, the wavelength of the light is measured with a sodium D-ray(589.3 nm). When the temperature is t ℃, the optical rotation is called the specific rotation of the substance, indicate as $[\alpha]_D^t$.

The specific rotation of glucose is +52.750°. Therefore, the polarimetry of glucose solution can be determined.

3　Instruments and Reagents

3.1　Instruments

100 mL volumetric flask, polarimeter, Nessler tube, arsenic test bottle, flat weighing bottle, drying oven, crucible, Muffle furnace, dryer, electronic balance.

3.2　Reagents

Ethanol, ammonia TS, alkaline cupric tartrate TS, phenolphthalein IS, sodium hydroxide VS, standard cobaltous chloride CS, standard potassium dichromate CS, standard copper sulfate CS, iodine TS, sulfosalicylic acid solution, diluted nitric acid, sodium chloride solution, silver nitrate solution, hydrochloric acid, potassium sulfate standard solution, barium chloride solution, ammonium thiocyanate solution, iron standard solution, lead standard solution, acetate buffer, thioacetamide test liquid, dilute sulfuric acid, potassium bromide-bromine TS, potassium iodide solution, acid tin chloride solution, arsenic standard solution, glucose, glucose injection, soluble starch.

4　Experimental Procedures

4.1　Description

Glucose is colorless crystal or white crystal or granular powder, odorless, sweet taste. Freely soluble in water and slightly soluble in ethanol.

Dissolve about 10 g of glucose, weighed accurately, with a quantity of water and 0.2 mL ammonia TS in a 100 mL volumetric flask and dilute with water to volume. Mix well and allow to stand for 10 min, the specific optical rotation of the resulting solution is +52.5° to +53.0°at 25 ℃.

4.2　Identification

(1) Dissolve about 0.2 g glucose in 5 mL of water, add dropwise hot alkaline cupric

tartrate TS; a red precipitate of cuprous oxide is produced.

(2) The infrared absorption spectrum is concordant with the following reference spectrum of glucose(Fig. 2 – 2 – 2).

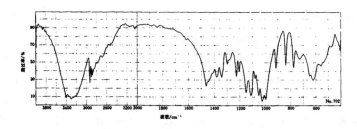

Fig. 2 –2 –2 Reference IR spectrum of glucose

4.3 Tests

4.3.1 Acidity

Dissolve 2. 0 g glucose in 20 mL of water, add 3 drops of phenolphthalein IS and 0. 20 mL of sodium of glucose(0. 02 mol/L) VS, a pink colour is produced.

4.3.2 Clarity and Colour of Solution

Dissolve 5 g glucose in hot water, cool, dilute to 10 mL with water, the solution is clear and colourless. Any opalescence produced is not more pronounced than that of reference suspension 1. Any colour produced is not more intense than that of a solution prepared by diluting 1. 0 mL of a reference solution(mix 3. 0 mL of standard cobaltous chloride CS and 3. 0 mL of standard potassium dichromate CS with 6. 0 mL of standard copper sulfate CS and add sufficient water to produce 50 mL) with water to 10 mL.

4.3.3 Clarify of Ethanoic Solution

Take 1. 0 g glucose add 20 mL of ethanol and reflux on a water bath for about 10 minutes, the solution is clear.

4.3.4 Sulfites and Soluble Starch

Dissolve 1. 0 g glucose in 10 mL of water, add 1 drop of iodine TS, a yellow colour is produced.

4.3.5 Loss on Drying

Take 1 ~ 2 g glucose, place it in a flat weighing bottle which is dried to constant weight under the same conditions as the sample. Make the sample spread flat on the bottom of the bottle with the thickness no more than 5 mm, add a cover and weigh it precisely. Put the weighing bottle in a clean culture dish, half-open the bottle cap or place it beside the bottle, and put it into a drying box at (105 ±2) ℃ for drying. Remove and quickly cover the bottle cap, place it in the dryer and cool it to room temperature, weigh the bottle quickly and accurately. When dried to constant weight at (105 ±2) ℃, it loses not less than 7. 5% and

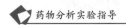

not more than 9. 5% of its weight.

4. 3. 6 Protein

Dissolve 1. 0 g glucose in 10 mL of water, add 3 mL of sulfosalicylic acid solution, no precipitate is produced.

4. 3. 7 Chlorides

Dissolve 0. 6 g glucose in 25 mL of water(if the solution is alkaline, it can be neutralized with nitric acid), add 10 mL of dilute nitric acid and filter if the solution is not clear. Place in 50 mL Nash tube, add water to make about 40 mL, shake well, and get the test solution. Place standard sodium chloride solution 6. 0 mL in another 50 mL Nessler tube, add water into about 40 mL, shake well, get the standard solution. In standard solution and test solution, add 1. 0 mL of silver nitrate solution, dilute with water to 50 mL, shake well. Allow to stand in the dark for 5 min, and compare the opalescence produced by viewing down the vertical axis of the cylinders against a black background. Any opalescent produced in the test solution is not more pronounced than that of the reference solution(0. 01%).

4. 3. 8 Sulfates

Dissolve 2. 0 g glucose in 40 mL of water in the 50 mL Nessler tube(if the solution is alkaline, it can be neutralized with hydrochloric acid) and filter if the solution is not clear. Add 2 mL of dilute hydrochloric acid, shake well, and get the test solution. Place standard potassium sulfate solution 2. 0 mL in another 50 mL Nessler tube, dissolved in water into 40 mL, dilute hydrochloric acid 2 mL, shake well, get the standard solution. In standard solution and test solution, add 5 mL 25% barium chloride solution, dilute with water to 50 mL, shake well, allow to stand in the dark for 10 min and compare the opalescence produced by viewing down the vertical axis of the cylinders against a black background. Any opalescent produced in the test solution is not more pronounced than that of the reference solution (0. 01%).

4. 3. 9 Iron

Dissolve 2. 0 g glucose in 20 mL of water, add 3 drop of nitric acid, boil gently for 5 min. Allow to cool, dilute to 45 mL with water, add 3 mL of ammonium thiocyanate solution, mix well. Any colour produced is not more intense than that of a reference solution prepared in the same manner using 2. 0 mL of iron standard solution(0. 01%).

4. 3. 10 Heavy Metals

Use two 50 mL Nessler tubes. Put a certain amount of standard lead solution and 2 mL acetate buffer(pH 3. 5) in tube A, dilute to 25 mL with water. Dissolve 4. 0 g glucose in 23 mL of water in tube B, add acetate buffer(pH 3. 5)2 mL. If the test solution is colored, drop a small amount of dilute caramel solution or other non-interference colored solution in tube A, make it consistent with tube B. And then add 2 mL of thioacetamide solution in two tubes, shake well, allow to stand for two minutes, compare the colour produced by viewing down the vertical axis of the cylinders against a white background, the color produced in the cylinder B is not more pronounced than that of the cylinder A(5 ppm).

4.3.11 Arsenic

Dissolve 2.0 g glucose in 5 mL of water, add 5 mL of dilute sulfuric acid and 0.5 mL of potassium bromide-bromine TS. Heat on a water bath for about 20 min and maintain the presence of excess of bromine. Add a quantity of potassium bromide-bromine TS, if necessary. Replace the evaporated water constantly and cool, then add 5 mL of hydrochloric acid and dilute with water to 28 mL. Add 5 mL potassium iodide solution and 5 drops of the acid tin chloride solution. Allow to stand at the room temperature for 10 min, add 2 g of zinc granules and quickly plug the bottle stopper(the test tube has cotton with lead acetate and the test paper of $HgBr_2$ placed on the bottle stopper). Heat on a water bath for about 45 min at 25~40 ℃. Take out the test paper of $HgBr_2$, any stain produced is not more intense than that of the standard stain(0.000 1%).

Arsenic standard stain place 2 mL of standard arsenic solution (1 μg/mL), accurately measured in another flask. Add 21 mL of water and 5 mL of hydrochloric acid, operate according to the above method.

4.3.12 Residue on Ignition

Place 1.0~2.0 g glucose in the crucible which previously ignited to constant weight, accurately weigh. Heat gently until it is thoroughly charred, cool it to the room temperature and moisten the residue with 0.5~1.0 mL of sulfuric acid. Heat gently until white fumes are no longer evolved and then ignite at 700~800 ℃ to constant weight. Put it in the dryer, cool to room temperature, accurately weigh, the residue on ignition should not exceed 0.1%.

4.4 Assay

Transfer an appropriate amount of glucose injection(equivalent to 10 g glucose), measured accurately, with a quantity of water and 0.2 mL of ammonia TS in a 100 mL volumetric flask and dilute with water to volume. Mix well(injections of 10% strength or less may be used directly without the addition of ammonia TS), allow to stand for 10 min.

Take out the measuring tube of the polarimeter and flush it several times with the test solution. Slowly load proper amount of the test solution(be careful not to cause bubbles). After cover sealing, place it in a polarimeter and slowly rotate the polarizer to check it until it looks uniform and bright. The degree expressed on the dial is the optical rotation of the test solution. Defining that the polarized light rotates to the right(clockwise) is called dextral, represented by the sign " + ", and the polarized light rotates to the left(counter clockwise) is called levorotation, represented by the sign " - ". Use the same method to measure the optical rotation at least 3 times and calculate the average value of them.

Set the reading of distilled water using the same method as blank. The observed rotation degree multiplied by 2.085 2, represents the weight of $C_6H_{12}O_6 \cdot H_2O$ in the test solution.

The Pharmacopoeia stipulates that glucose ($C_6 H_{12} O_6 \cdot H_2 O$) should be 95.0% to 105.0% of the labelled amount.

5 Precautions

(1) Colorimetric or turbidimetric operations should normally be performed in Nessler tubes. The volume of the sample tube is equal to that of the standard tube, the color of glass is same with the uniform scale. The difference should not be more than 2 mm.

(2) The operation of sample solution and reference solution should follow the principle of parallel operation, and attention should be paid to adding various reagents in order of operation.

(3) Before colorimetry and turbidimetry, the reagents in the colorimetric tube should be mixed well, and then the two tubes should be placed on the black or white background, and observed from top to bottom.

(4) In the arsenic analysis, the sample tube and the reference tube should be the same stress with the same length and the same inner diameter of the tube, so as to avoid the different size of the color spots, affecting the colorimetry. After the addition of zinc particles, the arsenic test tube should be covered and pressed immediately to avoid AsH_3 gas escaping.

(5) The operating conditions of constant weight such as the dryer used, the time of the crucible placed in the dryer, etc., must be consistent during determination of residue on ignition.

(6) When measuring the pH value, the electrode should be washed thoroughly with purified water before replacing the standard buffer or test solution, and then suck out the water. The standard buffer or test solution can also be used for washing. That the water is used to prepare the standard buffer and dissolve the sample should be cold distilled water with a pH of 5.5 ~ 7.0.

(7) The polarimeter should be preheated for 5 ~ 20 min after switching on the power. Before and after each test, the solvent is used for blank correction. When preparing and determining the solution, the temperature should be adjusted to (20 ± 0.5) ℃ (except otherwise specified). The test solution should be clarified. If it is turbid or contains suspended particles, it should be filtered at first and the primary filtrate is discarded. When the rotator is installed, attention should be paid to the absence of air bubbles in the optical path. After use, it should be washed and dried with water immediately. Do not use a brush, nor can it be baked at high temperature.

(8) Labelled amount, that is, specification or recipe quantity, represents the amount of the main drug contained in the unit preparation (for example, each tablet, pill, milliliter, bottle, etc.).

6 Questions

(1) What are the proposes of drug identification and test? What is the usual item of drug

tests?

(2) What are the standard operation procedures for the clarify test?

(3) How much of the lead standard solution should be taken for the limit test for heavy metals in this experiment according to the limit in glucose and the concentration of the standard lead solution?

(4) What precautions should be taken for the limit test for As(0822, method 1)? What is the function for each of the test solution added?

(5) Figure out the amount of the As standard solution that should be taken for the limit test for As(0822, method 1)(0.000 1%) in this experiment with the specified quantity of 2.0 g of sample.

(6) What does"ignite or dry to constant weight"mean? What is the key point during the determination of residue on ignition?

(7) Why is it necessary to use a tray balance to weigh a sample and a precision balance to weigh a crucible in the general impurity test of a drug?

(8) Can the limit test for As(0822, method 1) apply to all kinds of drugs? Why?

(9) Why do we check 5-hydroxymethyl furfural in glucose injection?

(10) What are the characteristics of the complete test of injection?

(11) When measuring the specific rotation of the glucose raw material by optical rotation method, why is it necessary to add ammonia TS and place it for the determination? When measuring the specific rotation with 10% glucose injection, why is it not necessary to add ammonia TS?

(12) Figure out the coefficient of 2.085 2 in the calculation of the glucose content in the assay of glucose by the method of optical rotation.

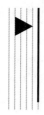

实验三 苯甲酸钠的分析

一、目的要求

（1）掌握钠盐及苯甲酸钠的鉴别方法。

（2）掌握双相滴定法的原理及操作。

（3）正确使用分液漏斗。

二、实验原理

钠盐燃烧在可见光区呈特异性鲜黄色，可用于鉴别。钠盐的中性溶液与醋酸氧铀锌试液作用，生成黄色醋酸氧铀锌钠结晶沉淀。

苯甲酸盐在中性溶液中与三氯化铁反应生成赭色碱式苯甲酸铁沉淀，加稀盐酸，赭色沉淀分解，游离出白色苯甲酸沉淀。苯甲酸盐与硫酸作用，析出具升华性的苯甲酸。

苯甲酸钠易溶于水，其水溶液为碱性，可用盐酸滴定液滴定。但滴定产物游离苯甲酸不溶于水，妨碍正确判断滴定终点。因此，加入乙醚，将苯甲酸提取至有机相，使其不干扰水相的滴定。

三、实验仪器与试剂

（一）仪器

分析天平、试管、分液漏斗、具塞锥形瓶、称量瓶、铂丝。

（二）试剂

醋酸氧铀锌试液、三氯化铁、稀盐酸、硫酸、乙醚、甲基橙指示剂、盐酸滴定液（0.5 mol/L）。

四、实验步骤

（一）鉴别

1. 钠盐

（1）取铂丝，用盐酸湿润后，蘸取本品在无色火焰中燃烧，火焰即显鲜黄色[《中国药典》（2020 年版）通则 0301]。

（2）取本品约 0.5 g，加水 10 mL 溶解，加酸调至中性后，加醋酸氧铀锌试液，即生成黄色沉淀。

2. 苯甲酸盐

（1）取本品约 0.5 g，加水 10 mL 溶解，加酸调至中性后，加三氯化铁试液，即生成赭色沉淀；加稀盐酸，变为白色沉淀。

（2）取本品适量，置干燥试管中，加硫酸后加热，不炭化，但析出苯甲酸，在试管内壁凝结成白色升华物。

（二）含量测定

取本品约 1.5 g，精密称定，置分液漏斗中，加水 25 mL，乙醚 50 mL 与甲基橙指示剂 2 滴，用盐酸滴定液（0.5 mol/L）滴定，边滴边振摇，至水层显橙红色；分取水层，置具塞锥形瓶中，乙醚层用水 5 mL 洗涤，洗液并入锥形瓶中，加乙醚 20 mL，继续用盐酸滴定液（0.5 mol/L）滴定，边滴边振摇，至水层显持续的橙红色，每 1 mL 盐酸滴定液（0.5 mol/L）相当于 72.06 mg 的 $C_7H_5NaO_2$。药典规定本品按干燥品计算，含 $C_7H_5NaO_2$ 不得少于 99.0%。

五、注意事项

（1）钠的火焰试验，最低检测限度约为 0.1 ng Na，若由试药和所用仪器引入微量钠盐时，均能出现鲜黄色火焰，故应在测试前将铂丝烧红，趁热浸入盐酸中，如此反复处理，直至火焰不显黄色，再蘸试样进行试验，且只有当强烈的黄色火焰持续数秒不退，才能确认为正反应。

（2）分液漏斗用前检漏，提取振摇时宜倾斜分液漏斗 150°，并不时排气。

（3）为了防止先加样品后加水的操作会使样品积聚在分液漏斗底部而不易全部溶解，可于分液漏斗中先加水，再加样品。

（4）双相滴定操作的关键是滴定速度要慢，振摇要充分，尤其近终点时，每加 1 滴均应充分振摇，以保证在二相间达到平衡。

（5）滴定反应终点偏酸性，故不能选酚酞为指示剂，应选择在酸性条件下变色的指示剂甲基橙。

六、思考题

（1）除了用甲基橙指示剂指示终点，还可采用什么方法判断终点？

（2）双相滴定适用于哪些药物的定量分析？

（3）双相滴定操作的关键是什么？如果振摇不充分会出现什么现象？为什么？

（4）双相滴定操作中，有哪些平行原则需要遵循？

（5）苯甲酸钠的含量测定采用盐酸标准溶液直接滴定的方法有什么缺点？

（6）苯甲酸钠、阿司匹林与三氯化铁的呈色反应是否相同？

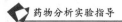

Experiment 3　The Analysis of Sodium Benzoate

1　Purposes

(1) To practice the identification method of the sodium salt and sodium benzoate.

(2) To master the principle and operation of the diphasic titration.

(3) To learn the correct use of the separatory funnel.

2　Principles

A bright yellow is presented in the visible region when sodium salt is burning, which can be used for identification. The neutral solution of sodium salt can react with uranium acetate zinc solution to form the yellow crystal precipitation of zinc acetate sodium.

Benzoate reacts with ferric chloride in neutral solution to form ochre basic ferric benzoate precipitate, dilute hydrochloric acid is added, ochre precipitate is decomposed, and white benzoic acid precipitate is separated. Benzoate is combined with sulfuric acid to produce sublimated benzoic acid. Sodium benzoate is easily soluble in water, and its aqueous solution is alkaline. It can be titrated by hydrochloric acid titrant. However, the free benzoic acid in the titration product is insoluble in water and hinders the correct judgement of titration end-point. Therefore, by adding ethyl ether, the benzoic acid is extracted to the organic phase, so that it do not interfere with the titration of the aqueous phase.

3　Instruments and Reagents

3.1　Instruments

Analytical balance, test tube, separatory funnel, stoppered conical flask, weighing bottle, platium wire.

3.2　Reagents

Uranyl zinc acetate test solution, ferric chloride solution, dilute hydrochloric acid, sulfuric acid, ether, methyl orange indicator, hydrochloric acid volumetric solution(VS) (0.5 mol/L)

4　Experimental Procedures

4.1　Identification

4.1.1　Sodium Salt

(1) Moisten sodium benzoatewith hydrochloric acid on a platinum wire, it imparts an intense yellow colour in a nonluminous flame(0301).

(2) Dissolve 0.5 g of sodium benzoate in 10 mL water, add uranyl zinc acetate test solution after adding acid to neutral, yellow precipitate is formed.

4.1.2　Benzoate

(1) Dissolve 0.5 g of sodium benzoate in 10 mL water, add acid to neutral, then add

ferric chloride TS, a dull yellow precipitate is formed which turns to white precipitate on addition of dilute hydrochloric acid.

(2) Introduce a quantity of sodium benzoate into a drying test tube, add sulfuric acid and heat gently, no charring occurs, a white sublimate of benzoic is deposited on the inner wall of the test tube.

4.2 Determination

Take about 1.5 g of sodium benzoate, weigh accurately, put it in a separatory funnel before 25 mL of water is added, then add 50 mL of ether and methyl orange indicator 2 drops. Titrate it with hydrochloric acid VS (0.5 mol/L), shake with the drop until the water layer shows the colour as orange red. Separate and place the water layer in a conical flask with plug. Wash the ether layer with 5 mL water, and washings also be placed into the conical flask. Add 20 mL of ether, and then the titration is continued with hydrochloric acid VS (0.5 mol/L), until an orange-red color is produced in the water layer and persists for several minutes. Each mL of hydrochloric acid (0.5 mol/L) is equivalent to 72.06 mg $C_7H_5NaO_2$. The Pharmacopoeia stipulates the content of sodium benzoate is not less than 99.0% of $C_7H_5NaO_2$ (calculated on the dried basis).

5 Precautions

(1) In the flame test of sodium, the minimum detection limit is about 0.1 ng Na. If the trace sodium salt is introduced into the test medicine and the instrument used, the bright yellow flame can appear. Therefore, the platinum wire should be burned red before the test, soaked in hydrochloric acid while hot, and treated repeatedly until the flame does not show yellow, and then dipped in the sample for testing, and only when intense yellow flames last for several seconds can they be identified as positive reactions.

(2) Take leak checking before using the separating funnel. When shaking to extract, the separation funnel should tilt 150° and exhaust from time to time.

(3) In order to prevent the sample from accumulating at the bottom of the separating funnel and not easy to dissolve completely, water can be added to the separating funnel first and then the sample is added.

(4) The key point of the two-phase titration is that the titration speed should be slow, shaking should be enough, especially near the end point, each drop should be added to shake fully to ensure that the balance between the two phases.

(5) The end point of titration reaction is acidic, so phenolphthalein cannot be chosen as an indicator. It is necessary to choose the methyl orange indicator in the acid condition.

6 Questions

(1) What other methods can be used to determine the end point except using methyl orange indicator to indicate the end point?

(2) What kind of drug is suitable for the quantitative analysis with two phase titration?

(3) What is the key point of the operation of titration reaction? What will happen if the shaking is not enough? Why?

(4) What parallel principles should we follow in the operation of titration reaction?

(5) What are the disadvantages of the direct titration of hydrochloric acid standard solution for the determination of sodium benzoate?

(6) Is the color of sodium benzoate reacting with ferric chloride the same as that of aspirin?

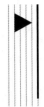

实验四 药物中特殊杂质的检查

一、目的与要求

（1）掌握药物特殊杂质的来源和检查原理。

（2）掌握薄层色谱法用于特殊杂质检查的一般操作。

（3）掌握薄层色谱中比移值（R_f）的计算方法。

二、实验原理

（一）阿司匹林中水杨酸的检查

水杨酸及其盐类在中性或弱酸性条件下，可与三氯化铁试液反应，生成紫色配位化合物。阿司匹林在生产过程中，可能存在水杨酸乙酰化不完全或贮藏过程中水解产生水杨酸。水杨酸可在弱酸性溶液中与高铁盐反应呈紫堇色，而阿司匹林结构中无游离酚羟基，不发生该反应，因而对杂质的检出无干扰。一定量水杨酸对照液在相同条件下与高铁盐反应，通过色泽比较，控制游离水杨酸的含量。化学反应式如下：

$$6 \begin{array}{c}\text{COOH}\\\text{——OH}\end{array} + 4Fe^{3+} \longrightarrow \left[Fe\left(\begin{array}{c}\text{COO}^-\\\text{——O}^-\end{array}\right)_2\right]_3 Fe + 12H^+$$

（二）氢化可的松中其他甾体的检查

甾体激素药物多由其他甾体化合物经结构改造而来，有关物质主要是药物中存在的合成起始物、中间体、副产物及降解产物等。由于这些杂质一般具有甾体的母核，和药物的结构相似，因此常采用色谱法进行检查，如薄层色谱法、高效液相色谱法等。

薄层色谱法（TLC）分离效能高，简便、快速，在有关物质检查中应用广泛。由于多数杂质是未知的，或是不稳定的，很难得到对照品，考虑到甾体激素类药物中的杂质多与药物结构相似，因此各国药典多采用自身稀释对照法进行检查，即用供试品溶液的稀释液作为对照，检查有关物质。供试品中的杂质经薄层色谱与药物分离后，其颜色与对照品溶液的主斑点比较，颜色不得更深。

氢化可的松为皮质激素类药物，C17 位上有 α 上醇酮基，具有还原性，能与具有氧化性的碱性四氮唑蓝反应，C17 位上的 α 上醇酮基被还原为红色的甲臜，此反应除用于显色鉴别试验外，还应用于皮质激素类药物薄层色谱的显色及含量测定等。

TLC 检查其他甾体的特点：①简便易行，不需要特殊的仪器；②不需要对照品；③只能控制单个杂质的限量；④要求杂质与主成分的显色灵敏度接近。

（三）肾上腺素中酮体的检查

肾上腺素在生产中均由其酮体氢化还原制成，若氢化不完全，易引入酮体杂质，因此《中国药典》规定检查酮体。肾上腺素与肾上腺酮的化学结构见图 2 - 4 - 1，其紫外吸收光谱图见图 2 - 4 - 2。从紫外吸收光谱图可见肾上腺酮在 310 nm 有最大吸收，而肾上腺素在此波长处无吸收，刚好可避开干扰，据此可通过紫外分光光度法直接测定肾上腺素中的杂质肾上腺酮且具有很好的专属性。

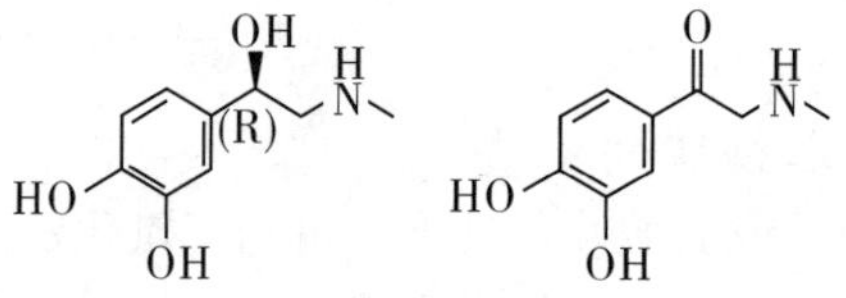

图 2 - 4 - 1　肾上腺素（A）与肾上腺酮（B）化学结构

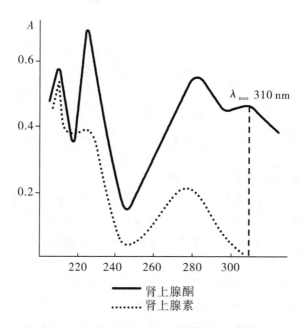

图 2 - 4 - 2　肾上腺素与肾上腺酮的紫外吸收光谱

（四）葡萄糖注射液中 5 - 羟甲基糠醛的检查

5 - 羟甲基糠醛（5-HMF）是葡萄糖等单糖化合物在高温或弱酸等条件下脱水产生的一个醛类化合物，对人体横纹肌和内脏有损害。该化合物稳定性不好，容易分解成乙酰丙酸和甲酸，或发生聚合反应。葡萄糖注射液在高温加热灭菌时易产生 5-HMF，其量的增加与灭菌温度、时间成正比，葡萄糖注射液在高温情况下颜色容易变黄，虽然 5-HMF 本身无色，但由于 5-HMF 可发生聚合而因聚合物导致变色，且葡萄糖注射液颜色的深浅与 5-HMF 产生的量成正比，因此，5-HMF 的量可指代产品中葡萄糖的分解程度。由于 5-HMF 的毒性及对产品质量的指示作用，在含葡萄糖或其他单糖的制剂中需要作为一个重要的指标加以控制。另外，在贮藏过程中，5-HMF 也会增加，因此应尽量缩短葡萄糖注射液的贮藏时间。

葡萄糖注射液颜色的深浅与 5-HMF 产生的量成正比，可通过控制溶液的颜色来控制 5-HMF 的量，但由于 5-HMF 并非葡萄糖注射液变色的唯一因素，该法专属性和准确性较差。5-HMF 的最大吸收波长为 284 nm，该处干扰较少，UV 法常可以作为 5-HMF 检查的首选方法。

三、实验仪器与试剂

（一）仪器

分析天平、硅胶 G 薄层板、层析缸、干燥箱、分光光度计、点样毛细管。

（二）试剂

乙醇、稀硫酸铁铵溶液、冰醋酸、氯仿、甲醇、二氯甲烷、乙醚、碱性四氮唑蓝试液、盐酸溶液、阿司匹林、水杨酸、氢化可的松、肾上腺素、葡萄糖注射液、三氯化铁试液。

四、实验步骤

（一）阿司匹林中水杨酸的检查

取本品 0.10 g，加乙醇 1 mL 溶解后，加冷水适量至 50 mL，立即加新制的稀硫酸铁铵溶液［取盐酸溶液（9→100）1 mL，加硫酸铁铵指示液 2 mL 后，再加水适量使成 100 mL］1 mL，摇匀；30 s 内若显色，与对照液（精密称取水杨酸 0.1 g，加水溶解后，加冰醋酸 1 mL，摇匀，再加水至 1 000 mL，摇匀，精密量取 1 mL，加乙醇 1 mL、水 48 mL 与上述新制的稀硫酸铁铵溶液 1 mL，摇匀）比较，颜色不得更深（0.1%）。

（二）氢化可的松中其他甾体的检查

取本品，加氯仿 - 甲醇（9∶1）制成每 1 mL 中含 6.0 mg 的溶液，作为供试品溶液；精密量取适量，加氯仿 - 甲醇（9∶1）稀释制成每 1 mL 中含 120 μg 的溶液，作为对照溶液。照薄层色谱法［《中国药典》（2020 年版）通则 0502］试验，吸取上述两种溶液各 10 μL，分别点于同一硅胶 G 薄层板上，以二氯甲烷 - 乙醚 - 甲醇 - 水（385：60：30：2）为展开剂，展开后，晾干，在 105 ℃干燥 10 min，放冷，喷以碱性四氮唑蓝试液，立即检视。供试品溶液若显杂质斑点，不得多于 3 个，其颜色与对照溶液的主斑点比较，颜色不得更深。

（三）肾上腺素中酮体的检查

取本品，加盐酸溶液（9→2 000）制成每 1 mL 中含 2.0 mg 的溶液，照分光光度法［《中国药典》（2020 年版）通则 0401］在 310 nm 的波长处测定，吸光度不得超过 0.05（酮体的吸收系数为 435）。

（四）葡萄糖注射液中 5 - 羟甲基糠醛的检查

精密量取葡萄糖注射液适量（约相当于葡萄糖 0.25 g），置 25 mL 量瓶中，用水稀释至刻度，摇匀，照 UV 法［《中国药典》（2020 年版）通则 0401］，在 284 nm 的波长处测定，吸光度不得超过 0.32。

五、注意事项

（1）点样采用微量毛细管进行，在距薄层板底边 2.0 cm 处开始，点样应少量多次点于同一原点处，原点面积应尽量小。

（2）采用倾斜上行法展开，展开剂应浸入薄层板底边约 1 cm 深度。

（3）碱性四氮唑蓝试液应临用新配，新鲜试剂应呈黄色，颜色若变深者不宜使用。

（4）显色后，应立即检视斑点，并用针头定位，以便记录图谱。

（5）游离水杨酸的检查样品应尽量干燥，不得带入过多水分，否则样品加醇后不易溶解。

（6）从展开缸中取出薄层板后应立即画出溶剂前沿，以免溶剂挥发后看不到溶剂前沿。

六、思考题

（1）薄层色谱法检查氢化可的松中其他甾体的原理是什么？为何用稀释液作为对照？

（2）试计算阿司匹林中游离水杨酸、氢化可的松中其他甾体、肾上腺素中酮体的杂质限度。

（3）试计算氢化可的松主斑点的比移值。

参考文献

[1] 国家药典委员会. 阿司匹林［M］//中华人民共和国药典（2010 年版二部）. 北京：中国医药科技出版社，2010：384.

［2］国家药典委员会. 氢化可的松［M］//中华人民共和国药典（2010 年版二部）. 北京：中国医药科技出版社，2010：550.

［3］国家药典委员会. 肾上腺素［M］//中华人民共和国药典（2010 年版二部）. 北京：中国医药科技出版社，2010：459.

［4］国家药典委员会. 葡萄糖注射液［M］//中华人民共和国药典（2010 年版二部）. 北京：中国医药科技出版社，2010：1516.

Experiment 4   The Tests of Specified Impurities in Drugs

1   Purposes

(1) To master the source and principle of the specified impurities in drugs.

(2) To master the general operation of TLC for specified impurities examination.

(3) To master the calculation method for R_f value in thin layer chromatography.

2   Principles

2.1   Detection of Salicylic Acid in Aspirin

Under neutral or weak acid condition, salicylic acid and its salts can react with ferric chloride solution to form purple coordination compounds. In the production of aspirin, there may be incomplete acetylation of salicylic acid or hydrolyed salicylic acid during the storage process. Salicylic acid can react with ferrate in weak acid solution as purple cordier, but there is no free phenolic hydroxyl in aspirin structure, so there is no interference to the detection of impurity. The content of free salicylic acid is controlled by reacting with ferrate under the same conditions as a certain amount of salicylic acid control solution(comparing the color).

2.2   Detection of Other Steroids In Hydrocortisone

Steroidal hormone drugs are mostly derived from other steroids through structural modification, and the related substances are mainly the synthetic starting materials, intermediates, by-products and degradation products. Because these impurities generally have the parent nucleus of steroids, which are similar with the structure of drugs, they are often examined by chromatography, such as thin layer chromatography, high performance liquid chromatography, etc.

Thin layer chromatography(TLC) has high separation efficiency, which is simple, fast and widely used in the test of related substances. Because most impurities are unknown or unstable, it is difficult to obtain the reference substance. Considering that the impurities in steroidal hormone drugs are mostly similar with the drug structure, pharmacopoeia in various countries mostly use self-controlled method for inspection, that is, the diluted test solution is used as the reference for inspection to check the related substances. After the impurities in the test sample are separated from the drug by TLC, their color shall not be deeper than that of the main spot of the control solution.

Hydrocortisone is a kind of corticosteroid drugs with an α-alcohol ketone group at the C17 position, which is reductive and can react with basic tetrazolium blue with oxidation. The α-alcohol ketone group at the C17 position is reduced to red formazan. This reaction is not only used for the color identification test, but also used for the color development and content determination of corticosteroids by thin-layer chromatography.

The characteristics of TLC test of other steroid are as follows: ①It is simple and easy to be operated, no special equipment is required. ②No reference substance is required. ③It is only used for the limit of a single impurity. ④ The sensitivity of impurities and main components should be close.

2. 3 Examination of Ketones in Adrenaline

Adrenaline is produced by hydrogenation and reduction of its ketone body in the production. If hydrogenation is not complete, impurities of ketone body are easily introduced, so it is required to check ketone body in *Chinese Pharmacopoeia*. The chemical structure of adrenaline and adrenalone is shown in Fig. 2 – 4 – 1; and its UV absorption spectrum is shown in Fig. 2 – 4 – 2. It can be seen from the ultraviolet absorption spectrum that adrenalone has the maximum absorption at 310 nm, while adrenaline has no absorption at this wavelength, just avoiding interference. Therefore, the impurity adrenalone in adrenaline can be directly determined by UV spectrophotometry with good specificity.

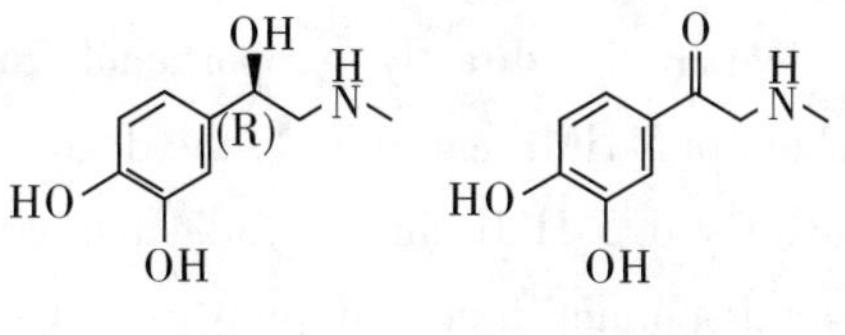

Fig. 2 –4 –1　Chemical structure of adrenaline(A) and adrenalone(B)

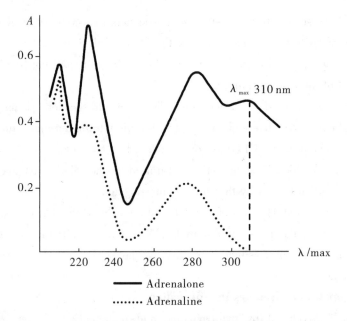

Fig. 2 −4 −2   Ultraviolet absorption spectrum of adrenaline and adrenalone

2. 4   Detection of 5-Hydroxymethyl Furfural in Glucose Injection

5-hydroxymethyl Furfural (5-HMF) is an aldehyde compound produced by the dehydration of monosaccharide compounds such as glucose under the conditions of high temperature or weak acid, which damages the human striated muscle and internal organs. It is easy to be decomposed into levulinic acid and formic acid, or polymerize. Glucose injection is easy to produce 5-HMF when it is heated and sterilized at high temperature. The increase of 5-HMF is directly proportional to sterilization temperature and time. The color of glucose injection is easy to turn yellow under high temperature. Although 5-HMF itself is colorless, the color of glucose injection is changed by polymer due to polymerization of 5-HMF, and the color depth of glucose injection is directly proportional to the amount of 5-HMF produced. Therefore, the amount of 5-HMF can refer to the degree of decomposition of glucose in the product. Due to the toxicity of 5-HMF and its indicative effect on product quality, it is necessary to control it as an important index in preparations containing glucose or other monosaccharides. In addition, 5-HMF will increase during storage, so the storage time of glucose injection should be shortened as much as possible.

Because the color depth of glucose injection is directly proportional to the amount of 5-HMF produced, the amount of 5-HMF can be controlled by controlling the color of the solution, but because 5-HMF is not the only factor causing the discoloration of glucose injection, the specificity and accuracy of this method are poor. The maximum absorption wavelength of 5-HMF is 284 nm, where there is less interference. UV method can often be used as the first choice for 5-HMF detection.

3　Instruments and Reagents

3.1　Instruments

Analytical balance, silica gel G thin layer plate, chromatography cylinder, drying oven, UV spectrometer, microcap.

3.2 Reagents

Ethanol, dilute ammonium ferric sulfate solution, glacial acetic acid, chloroform, methanol, dichloromethane, diethyl ether, basic tetrazolium blue test solution, hydrochloric acid solution, aspirin, salicylic acid, hydrocortisone, adrenaline, glucose injection, ferric chloride test solution.

4　Experimental Procedures

4.1　Examination of Salicylic Acid in Aspirin

Dissolve 0.10 g of aspirin in 1 mL of ethanol, add cold water to 50 mL, then immediately add 1 mL of freshly prepared dilute ferric ammonium sulfate solution(to 1 mL of 1 mol/L hydrochloric acid solution, add 2 mL of ferric ammonium sulfate TS and add water to volume of 100 mL), and mix well; any colour produced in 30 s is not more intense than that of a reference solution(Dissolve 0.1 g of salicylic acid, accurately measured, in water and then add 1 mL of glacial acetic acid, mix well; add water to produce 1 000 mL, mix well. To 1 mL of the solution, accurately measured, add 1 mL of ethanol, 48 mL of water and 1 mL of the freshly prepared dilute ferric ammonium sulfate solution above, mix well)(0.1%).

4.2　Determination of Other Steroids in Hydrocortisone Acetate

Dissolve a quantity of hydrocortisone acetate in mixture of chloroform-methanol (9:1) to produce a solution containing 6.0 mg/mL as the test solution. Transfer a quantity of the test solution in mixture of chloroform-methanol(9:1) to produce a solution containing 120 μg per mL as the reference solution. Carry out the method for thin-layer chromatography (General Rule 0502), using silica gel G as the coating substance and a mixture of dichloromethane-ether-methanol-water(385:60:30:2) as mobile phase. Apply separately to the plate 10 μL each of two solutions in chloroform-methanol(9:1) containing(1)3.0 mg per mL and(2)60 μg/mL of the substance being examined. After developing and removal of the plate, dry it in air, heat at 105 ℃ for 10 min, stand to room temperature, spray with alkaline tetrazolium blue TS, examine immediately. Any spot in the chromatogram obtained with solution(1) other than the principal spot is not more intense than the principal spot obtained with solution(2) and the number of spots is not more than 3.

4.3　Test of Adrenalone in Adrenaline

Dissolve a quantity of adrenaline in hydrochloric acid TS(9→2 000) to produce a solution containing 2.0 mg/mL. The absorbance should not exceed 0.05 measured by spectrophotometer

(General Rule 0401) at the wavelength of 310 nm(The absorption coefficient of adrenalone is 453 at 310 nm).

4.4 Test of 5-Hydroxymethyl Furfural in Glucose Injection

Measure accurately a volume equivalent to 0.25 g to a 25 mL volumetric flask, dilute with water to volume and mix well, measure the absorbance at 284nm(General Rule 0401) it, the absorbance is less than 0.32.

5 Precautions

(1)Sampling with micro-syringe should start at 2.0 cm away from the bottom of the thin-layer plate, a small number of points should be repeated at the same origin, and the origin area should be as small as possible.

(2)Using the upward sloping method, the developer should be immersed in the depth of 1 cm at the bottom edge of the thin plate.

(3)The alkaline tetrazolium blue test solution should be fresh when we use it with the colour as yellow, and the solution with darker color is not suitable for use.

(4)After staining, check the spots immediately and locate them with a needle to record the map.

(5)The sample of aspirin for free salicylic acid test should be as dry as possible, do not bring too much moisture, otherwise the sample is not easy to dissolve after adding alcohol.

(6)Draw the front edge of the solvent immediately after taking out the thin plate from the chromatographic tank, so as to avoid invisible of the front edge of the solvent due to the solvent volatilization.

6 Questions

(1)What is the principle of the TLC examining other steroids in hydrocortisone? Why use diluent solution as a control?

(2)Try to calculate the impurity limit of free salicylic acid in aspirin, other steroids in hydrocortisone and ketones in epinephrine.

(3)Try to calculate R_f value of the main spot of hydrocortisone.

References

[1] Chinese Pharmacopoeia Commission. Aspirin [M] //Chinese pharmacopoeia (2010 edition, Part Ⅱ). Beijing: China Medical Science Press, 2010: 384.

[2] Chinese Pharmacopoeia Commission. Hydrocortisone [M] //Chinese pharmacopoeia (2010 edition, Part Ⅱ). Beijing: China Medical Science Press, 2010: 550.

[3] Chinese Pharmacopoeia Commission. Adrenaline [M] //Chinese pharmacopoeia (2010 edition, Part Ⅱ). Beijing: China Medical Science Press, 2010: 459.

[4] Chinese Pharmacopoeia Commission. Glucose injection [M]//Chinese pharmacopoeia(2010 edition, Part Ⅱ). Beijing: China Medical Science Press, 2020: 1516.

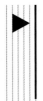

实验五　复方丹参滴丸中冰片、丹参的薄层色谱法分析

一、实验目的

（1）熟悉中药的鉴别方法。
（2）掌握复方丹参滴丸中冰片、丹参的薄层色谱鉴别法。
（3）掌握样品前处理的原理及方法。

二、实验原理

薄层色谱兼具分离与鉴别特性，并且具有直观、承载信息大、专属性强、快速、经济、操作简便等优点，是中药材及中成药鉴别的重要方法。中成药质量标准研究技术要求：①复方制剂的薄层鉴别药味应达到处方药味一半以上，首选君臣药、贵重药、易混淆药鉴别。②制剂中各药味的鉴别方法除前处理外，原则上应尽量与该药材和饮片的专属鉴别方法一致，若因其他成分干扰或制剂的提取方法不同，可采用其他鉴别方法。③尽可能采取一个供试液多项多维鉴别使用，达到节约资源、保护环境、简便实用的目的，同时系列品种其鉴别方法应保持一致。另外，要注重绿色环保要求，展开剂尽量采用毒害小、污染少的试剂与试药，避免使用苯等毒性大的溶剂，并尽量采用《中国药典》附录中已收载的试剂与试液。

遵循上述原则及规定，选用薄层色谱法时，应以图谱清晰、斑点明显、阴性无干扰、分离度符合要求（$R > 1.0$）、R_f 适中（$0.2 \sim 0.8$）、专属性强、重现性与耐用性符合要求等为评价指标；需要完成供试品制备方法考察、显色条件考察（如日光、紫外、显色剂），利用阴性空白试验证明其他药味无干扰，考察不同品牌薄层板、不同温度、湿度等条件下方法的耐用性。

丹参滴丸由丹参、三七和冰片组成，主要作用是活血化瘀、理气止痛，用于治疗胸中憋闷、心绞痛，其主要有效成分为丹参药材中的丹参酮 II A、隐丹参酮、丹参素、丹酚酸类等物质，三七药材中的三七皂苷 R_1、人参皂苷 R_{b1}、人参皂苷 R_{g1}、人参皂苷 R_e 等及冰片。本实验以中成药复方丹参滴丸中的冰片及丹参素成分为分析对象，超声提取其中的冰片，以天然冰片作为对照，在薄层色谱条件下进行鉴别；乙酸乙酯提取其中的丹参素，以丹参素钠为对照品，用薄层色谱鉴别复方丹参滴丸中的丹参。中药的鉴别目前以薄层色谱为主，常在对主要成分经提取、分离和纯化后，以对照品、对照药材或对照提取物作为定性的参考依据。

三、实验仪器与试剂

(一)仪器
超声波清洗机、硅胶 G 薄层板、层析缸、干燥箱、暗箱紫外分析仪。

(二)试剂
无水乙醇、环己烷、乙酸乙酯、三氯甲烷、丙酮、甲酸、1% 香草醛硫酸溶液、稀盐酸、冰片对照品、丹参素钠对照品、复方丹参滴丸。

四、实验步骤

(一)冰片的鉴别
取本品 20 丸,碾碎,加无水乙醇 5 mL,超声处理 10 min,滤过,滤液作为供试品溶液。另取冰片对照品,加无水乙醇制成每毫升含 1 mg 的溶液,作为对照品溶液。照薄层色谱法 [《中国药典》(2020 年版)通则 0502]试验,吸取上述两种溶液各 5~10 μL,分别点于同一硅胶 G 薄层板上,以环己烷 – 乙酸乙酯(17:3)为展开剂,展开,取出,晾干,喷以 1% 香草醛硫酸溶液,在 105 ℃ 加热至斑点显色清晰。供试品色谱中,在与对照品色谱相应的位置上,显相同颜色的斑点。

(二)丹参的鉴别
取本品 15 丸,置离心管中,加水 1 mL 和稀盐酸 2 滴,振摇使溶解,加入乙酸乙酯 3 mL,振摇 1 min 后离心 2 min,取上清液作为供试品溶液。另取丹参素钠对照品,加 75% 甲醇制成每 1 mL 含 1 mg 的溶液,作为对照品溶液。照薄层色谱法 [《中国药典》(2020 年版)通则 0502]试验,吸取供试品溶液 10 μL、对照品溶液 2 μL,分别点于同一硅胶 G 薄层板上,以三氯甲烷 – 丙酮 – 甲酸(25:10:4)为展开剂,展开,取出,晾干,置氨蒸气中熏 15 min 后,显淡黄色斑点,放置 30 min 后置紫外光(365 nm)下检视。供试品色谱中,在与对照品色谱相应的位置上,显相同颜色的荧光斑点。

五、注意事项

(1)点样:点样要少量多次,点样直径不超过 3 mm,点样距离一般为 1.0~1.5 cm 即可,点样量不可过多,防止超载,点样时必须注意勿损伤薄层表面,点样后必须将溶剂全部除去后再进行展开,但要避免高温加热,以免改变待测成分的性质。

(2)展开剂:注意每次展开时临用现配展开剂;小比例展开剂用移液管准确加入;当展开剂中有氨水时,若展开效果不好,应考虑氨水易挥发,用未开封的氨水重新配制展开剂。

(3)展开:相对湿度不同,分离效果不同;薄层板要在加有展开剂的层析缸中预饱和，防止边缘效应；温度会影响展开效果，有时温度降低，改善分离效果；展距过长，斑点扩散，过短，分离效果不好；展开缸应相对应。10 cm×20 cm 的板就用 10 cm×20 cm 的展开缸；展开缸盖不宜用凡士林密闭，应为毛玻璃盖密封加重物。

（4）在加热显色时，不同的样品可能需要不同的温度、不同的时间，注意密切观察。

（5）显色剂要适量喷雾显色，注意使雾滴均匀；硫酸容易吸收水分，因此从显色完成到加热的过程的时间要控制得尽量短。

六、预习提要

（1）薄层色谱操作的步骤主要包括哪些？
（2）中药定性鉴别常用的标准物质有哪些？
（3）硫酸乙醇液应如何配制？
（4）中药制剂进行鉴别或含量测定时，被测成分选取的原则是什么？
（5）如何进行薄层色谱系统适应性试验？

七、思考题

（1）中药薄层色谱鉴别结果分析时需要注意哪些问题？
（2）为什么中药鉴别常采用薄层色谱法？
（3）薄层色谱法的系统适用性试验包括哪些内容？
（4）请分析复方丹参滴丸中冰片、丹参的 TLC 检查时样品前处理的目的和原理。

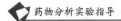

Experiment 5　TLC Analysis of Borneol and Salvia Miltiorrhiza in Compound Danshen Dripping Pills

1　Purposes

(1) To study the identification of Chinese herbal medicine.

(2) To master the TLC identification of salvia miltiorrhiza and borneol in compound Danshen dripping pills.

(3) To master the principle and method of the sample pretreatment.

2　Principles

TLC has the characteristics of separation and identification, and has the advantages of intuitive, large information, strong specificity, fast, economic, simple operation and so on. It is an important method for the identification of traditional Chinese medicine and Chinese patent medicine. The technical requirements for the quality standard research of Chinese patent medicine are as follows: ① The TLC identification of compound preparation should reach more than half of the kinds of herbal medicines in prescription, and the first choice is to identify main medicine and assistant medicine, precious medicine and easily confused medicine. ② The TLC identification of compound preparation should be based on the quality standard research of Chinese patent medicine except for pretreatment, the identification method of each herbs in the preparation should be consistent with the exclusive identification method of the medicinal material and decoction pieces as far as possible, and other identification methods can be used due to interference of other components or different extraction methods of the preparation. ③ Multi-dimensional identification of one test solution should be adopted as far as possible, so as to save resources and protect the environment, and achieve simple and practical purposes. The identification methods should be consistent for series products. In addition, we should pay attention to the requirements of green environmental protection, try to use reagents and test drugs with less toxicity and pollution, avoid using benzene and other toxic solvents, and try to use reagents and test solutions contained in the appendix of *Chinese Pharmacopoeia*.

In accordance with the above principles and regulations, the clear chromatogram, obvious spots, no negative interference, resolution meeting the requirements($R > 1.0$), moderate R_f value($0.2 \sim 0.8$), strong specificity, reproducibility and durability meeting the requirements should be taken as the evaluation indexes when selecting TLC. The preparation method of the test sample and the chromogenic conditions(such as sunlight, ultraviolet and chromogenic agent) should be investigated. The negative blank test is used to prove that there is no interference from other medicines, and the durability of different brands of TLC, different temperatures and humidity are should also be investigated.

Compound Danshen dripping pill is composed of salvia miltiorrhiza, panax notoginseng and borneol. Its main functions are promoting blood circulation and removing blood stasis, regulating Qi and relieving pain. In this experiment, the composition of borneol in the traditional Chinese medicine Danshen dropping pill is analyzed. The borneol is extracted by ultrasound, and then the borneol is identified by TLC with natural borneol as the control. Salvianic acid in compound Danshen dripping pills is extracted using ethyl acetate. Salvianic acid A sodium is used as the reference substances to identificate the salvia miltiorrhiza in pills by TLC. At present, the identification of traditional Chinese medicine is mainly based on TLC. After the extraction, separation and purification of the main components, the reference substances, the reference herbs or the reference extracts are usually taken as the qualitative basis.

3　Instruments and Reagents

3.1　Instruments

Ultrasonic cleaning machine, silica gel G thin layer plate, chromatography cylinder, drying oven, black box ultraviolet analyzer.

3.2　Reagents

Anhydrous ethanol, cyclohexane, ethyl acetate, chloroform, acetone, formic acid, 1% vanillin sulfuric acid solution, dilute hydrochloric acid, borneol RS, salvianic acid A sodium RS, compound Danshen dripping pill.

4　Experimental Procedures

4.1　Identification of Borneol

Take 20 pills, crush it, add 5 mL of anhydrous ethanol, and conduct ultrasonic treatment for 10 min, and filter the filtrate as the test solution. Take another borneol control sample and add anhydrous ethanol to make the solution containing 1 mg per mL as the control solution. Carry out the method for TLC(Generl Rule 0502). Apply separately to the plate coated with silica G 5 ～ 10 μL of each of the two solutions, using cyclohexane-ethyl acetate (17 : 3) as mobile phase. After developing and removal of the plate, allow it to the dry in air. Spray with 1% vanillin in sulfuric acid solution, heat at 105 ℃ until the spot color is clear. The colour and position of the spots in the chromatogram obtained with test solution corresponds to that of the spot due to borneol in the chromatogram obtained with the reference solution.

4.2　Identification of Salvia Miltiorrhiza

Put 15 pills into a centrifuge tube, add 1 mL of water and 2 drops of dilute hydrochloric acid, shake well, add 3 mL of ethyl acetate, shake them for 1 min and then centrifuge for 2 min, take the supernatant as the test solution. In addition, transfer a quantity of salvianic acid A sodium reference substance, add 75% methanol to make a solution containing 1 mg per mL as the reference solution. Carry out the method for TLC(General Rule 0502) , apply separately to the plate coated with silica G 10 μL of test solution and 2 μL of reference solution, using chloroform-acetone-formic acid(25 ∶ 10 ∶ 4) as the developing solvent. After developing and removal of the plate, allow it to the dry in air. Smoke the plate in ammonia, steam it for 15 min until the light yellow spots are display, then examine the plate under ultraviolet light(365 nm) after it is stood for 30 min. The colour and position of the spots in the chromatogram obtained with test solution corresponds to that of the spot due to salvianic acid A sodium in the chromatogram obtained with the reference solution.

5 Precautions

(1) Modes and techniques of sample application: Sampling should be small amount once and many times, the diameter of the sample should not be more than 3 mm, and the sampling distance should be 1. 0 ~ 1. 5 cm. The amount of sampling should not be too much to prevent overloading. Attention must be paid not to damage the surface of the thin layer when sampling. After sampling, the solvent must be completely removed before development. However, high temperature heating should be avoided to avoid changing the properties of the components to be tested.

(2) The preparation of developing solvent: Pay attention to the temporary use of ready-made developing agent each time; small proportion of developing agent should be accurately added by pipette; when there is ammonia in the developing agent, if the development effect is not good, it should be considered that the ammonia is easy to volatilize, and the unsealed ammonia should be used to prepare the development agent again.

(3) Development: the separation effect is different with different relative humidity. The thin layer plate should be presaturated in the chromatographic cylinder with developer to prevent edge effect. The development effect will be affected by temperature. Sometimes, decreasing temperature will improve the separation effect. If the developing distance is too long, the spot will diffuse; it is too short, the separation effect is not good. The chromatographic cylinder should correspond to the size of the thin plate. A 10 cm × 20 cm cylinder should be used for a 10 cm × 20 cm plate; the cylinder head should not be sealed with vaseline, but should be sealed with ground glass cover or adding a heavy object.

(4) Different samples may need different temperature and time during heating and color development. Closely observe the experimental phenomena.

(5) The appropriately amount of color reagent should be sprayed on the plate, pay attention to the uniform droplet. Sulfuric acid is easy to absorb moisture, so the process from color completion to heating should be controlled as short as possible.

6 Previews

(1) What are the main steps of TLC?

(2) What are the commonly used reference substances for the qualitative identification of traditional Chinese medicine?

(3) How to prepare the sulfuric acid ethanol solution?

(4) What is the principle for the selection as the marker when traditional Chinese medicine to be identified or determined?

(5) How to carry out the TLC system suitability test?

7 Questions

(1) What should be paid attention to when analyzing the results of TLC?

(2) Why TLC is often used in the identification for traditional Chinese medicine?

(3) What are the contents of the TLC system suitability test?

(4) Please analyze the purpose and principle of sample pretreatment in TLC examination of borneol and salvia miltiorrhiza in compound Danshen dropping pills.

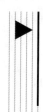

实验六　甘油磷酸钠含量测定

一、实验目的

（1）掌握电位滴定法的原理及操作。
（2）掌握电位滴定法确定终点的方法。
（3）掌握甘油磷酸钠含量测定和含量计算的方法。
（4）了解电位滴定法的应用及电极的选择。

二、实验原理

电位滴定法是根据滴定过程中电极电位的变化来确定滴定终点，计算待测物含量的分析方法，特别适用于化学反应平衡常数较小、滴定突跃不明显或试液有色、呈现浑浊的情况。

电位滴定的仪器装置如图2-6-1所示。试液中插入指示电极和参比电极构成工作电池，滴定过程不断测量工作电池电动势的变化，达化学计量点时，由于浓度的变化，引起指示电极电位突变，而使工作电池电动势发生突变，从而指示滴定终点的到达。本法可用于酸碱滴定、氧化还原滴定、沉淀滴定和配合物滴定。根据待测离子性质的不同，选用不同的指示电极和参比电极。

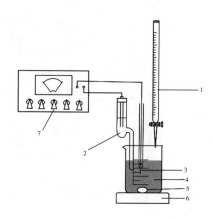

1. 滴定管；2. 参比电极；3. 指示电极；4. 待测溶液；5. 搅拌子；6. 电磁搅拌器；7. pH-mV电位测量仪。

图2-6-1　电位滴定装置

以 0.1 mol/L AgNO$_3$溶液滴定氯化钠溶液为例加以说明，滴定数据见表 2 – 6 – 1，滴定数据处理曲线见图 2 – 6 –2。

表 2 – 6 – 1　电位滴定部分数据

V/mL	E/mV	ΔE/mV	ΔV/mL	$\Delta E/\Delta V$ /（mV/mL）	$\bar{V}$/mL	$\Delta^2 E$	Δ（$\Delta E/\Delta V$）	$\Delta^2 E/\Delta V^2$
				…… ……				
10.00	168							
		34	1.00	34	10.50			
11.00	202							—
		16	0.20	80	11.10			
11.20	218							
		7	0.05	140	11.225			
11.25	225（$E1$）						120	2 400
		13（ΔE_1）	0.05	260	11.275			
11.30	238（$E2$）						280	5 600
		27（ΔE_2）	0.05	540	11.325	14（$\Delta^2 E_1$）		
11.35	265（$E3$）						−20	−400
		26（ΔE_3）	0.05	520	11.375	−1（$\Delta^2 E_2$）		
11.40	291（$E4$）						−220	4 400
		15	0.05	300	11.425			
11.45	306							—
		10	0.05	200	11.475			
11.50	316							
				…… ……				

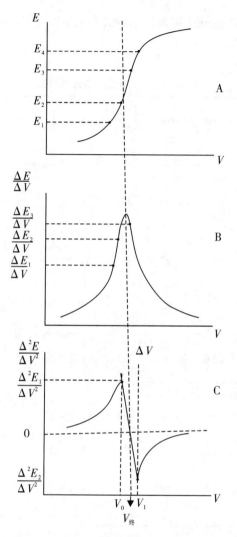

图2-6-2 0.1 mol/L AgNO₃ 溶液滴定氯化钠溶液的滴定数据处理曲线

从图2-6-2看，如果选用的 ΔV 足够小且相等，$\dfrac{\Delta^2 E}{\Delta V^2} \rightarrow \dfrac{\mathrm{d}^2 E}{\mathrm{d} V^2}$，滴定终点附近的曲线可近似地看作直线，所以二级微商法的终点根据相似三角形原则有：

$$\left| \frac{\Delta^2 E_1}{\Delta V^2} \right| \bigg/ \frac{\Delta E_2}{\Delta V^2} = \frac{V_{\text{终}} - V_0}{V_1 - V_{\text{终}}} \Rightarrow V_{\text{终}} = \frac{|\Delta^2 E_1| V_1 + |\Delta^2 E_2| V_0}{= |\Delta^2 E_1| + |\Delta^2 E_2|}$$

由于 $V_1 = V_0 + \Delta V$，$\Delta E_1 = E_2 - E_1$，$\Delta E_2 = E_3 - E_2$，$\Delta E_3 = E_4 - E_3$，$\Delta^2 E_1 = \Delta E_2 - \Delta E_1 = E_3 - 2E_2 + E_1$，$\Delta^2 E_2 = E_4 - 2E_3 + E_2$，所以：

$$V_{终} = V_0 + \frac{|\ E_3 - 2E_2 + E_1\ |\ \cdot \Delta V}{|\ E_3 - 2E_2 + E_1\ |\ +\ |\ E_4 - 2E_3 + E_2\ |}$$

通常采用以下三种方法确定终点：①$E-V$曲线法。以滴定体积（V）为横坐标，以电位计读数为纵坐标作图，得到一条S形曲线，见图2-6-2A。曲线的转折点（拐点）即为滴定终点，此法较方便，但要求滴定化学计量点处的突跃明显。②$\Delta E/\Delta V - V$曲线法。用表2-6-1中数据对平均体积（计算 ΔE 值时，前后两体积的平均值）作图，得一曲线，见图2-6-2B。峰状曲线的最高点所对应的体积即为滴定终点体积，该点的横坐标恰好与 $\Delta E/\Delta V - V - V$ 曲线的拐点横坐标重合，如图中竖直虚线所示。该法也叫一级微商法。③$\Delta^2 E/\Delta V^2 - V$ 曲线法。用表2-6-1中数据 $\Delta^2 E/\Delta V^2$ 对体积（V）作图，得到一条具有两个极值的曲线，如图2-6-2C所示，通常一级微商曲线的极大值为终点，则其二级微商必定等于零，此点也为终点，见图2-6-2C，该法又称二级微商法。由于滴定终点附近的曲线线段可近似地看作直线，因此，二级微商法的终点也可利用表2-6-1中数据，不用作图法而用内插法确定。

由此可见，与已知的终点计算方法相比，该方法具有推导简单、计算方便的特点，计算结果准确，化学计量点前后只需仔细读取少数数值。

甘油磷酸钠为 α-甘油磷酸二钠盐与 β-甘油磷酸二钠盐的混合物，按无水物计算，含 $C_3H_7Na_2O_6P$ 应为98.0%～102.0%。

甘油磷酸钠的结构如图2-6-3所示：

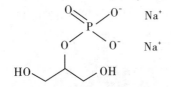

图2-6-3 甘油磷酸钠的结构

分子式：$C_3H_7Na_2O_6P \cdot 5H_2O$
分子量：306.11
不含水的分子量：216.11
含量测定反应：$2\ C_3H_7Na_2O_6P + H_2SO_4 = 2\ C_3H_7NaHO_6P + Na_2SO_4$
摩尔比：2:1
每毫升的硫酸滴定液（0.05 mol/L）相当于21.6 mg 的 $C_3H_7Na_2O_6P$。

三、实验仪器与试剂

（一）仪器
分析天平、电位滴定仪、10 mL 滴定管、玻璃电极、甘汞电极。

（二）试剂

硫酸滴定液（0.05 mol/L）、甘油磷酸钠、酚酞指示液。

四、实验步骤

取本品约 0.2 g，精密称定，加水 30 mL 溶解，加酚酞指示液 4 滴，用硫酸滴定液（0.05 mol/L）滴定至恰使溶液无色后，照电位滴定法 [《中国药典》（2020 年版）通则 0701]，用硫酸滴定液（0.05 mol/L）滴定。每 1 mL 硫酸滴定液（0.05 mol/L）相当于 21.6 mg 的 $C_5H_7N_2O_6P$。

上述操作的同时，在滴定液中，插入玻璃电极－甘汞电极，将其连到电位滴定装置上，观察并记录加入不同体积滴定液后的电位值。

此外，在滴定至近终点时，每加 0.10 mL 滴定液，记录一次电位值，用一阶求导或二阶导数法求出终点时所需滴定液的体积，计算含量。

五、注意事项

（1）滴定时电磁搅拌的速度不宜过快，以不产生空气旋涡为宜。

（2）要准确地记录滴定液的体积和电位值。

（3）滴定体积间隔不能过大，可以 1 滴（0.05 mL）进行。

（4）可先预估下含量，在接近终点附近开始等体积加入滴定液（98% ×分子量 $C_5H_7N_2O_6P$/分子量 $C_3H_7Na_2O_6P \cdot 5H_2O$ = 98% ×216.11/306.11 = 69.19%）。

六、思考题

（1）电位滴定法的特点是什么？

（2）如何减少电位测量的误差？

（3）用电位滴定法进行甘油磷酸钠含量测定时，为什么要先将供试液用硫酸滴定至酚酞无色？

（4）比较指示剂法与电位法指示终点的优缺点。

参考文献

[1] 国家药典委员会 . 中华人民共和国药典（2020 年版二部）[M].北京：中国医药科技出版社，2020：135.

[2] 徐新军 . 一种简单的计算电位滴定终点的方法 [J].广东药学，1997（3）：25 – 26.

Experiment 6　Assay of Sodium Glycerophosphate

1　Purposes

(1) To master the principle and operation of potentiometric titration.

(2) To master the potential method to determine the end point.

(3) To understand the assay of sodium glycerophosphate and the method to calculate its content.

(4) To understand where to use potentiometric titration and how to select electrode.

2　Principles

Potentiometric titration is a method to determine the titration end point and calculate the content of the substance to be measured according to the change of electrode potential in the process of titration, which is especially suitable for those that chemical reaction equilibrium constant is small, leap point is not obvious, or test solution is of color or appear turbidity.

The apparatus for potentiometric titration is shown in Fig. 2 − 6 − 1. The indicator electrode and the reference electrode are insered in test solution to form working battery, the change of the potential in the titration process is continuously measured. When reaching the stoichiometric point, the sudden change of the potential of the working battery happens owning to a sudden change of the potential of the indicator electrode caused by the change of the concentration, which indicates the arrival of the end point of the titration. This method can be used in acid-base titration, redox titration, precipitation titration and complex titration. The different indicator electrodes and reference electrodes are selected according to the different properties of the ions to be measured.

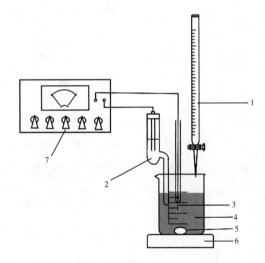

1. Burette; 2. Reference electrode; 3. Indicator electrode; 4. Test solution; 5. Stirrer; 6. Electromagnetic stirrer; 7. pH-mV meter.

Fig. 2 − 6 − 1　Potentiometric titration apparatus

Taking the data of titration of sodium chloride with 0. 1 mol/L AgNO₃ standard solution as an example to explain the above theory, the data of titration are shown in Tab. 2 − 6 − 1, and the curves of titration are shown in Fig. 2 − 6 − 2.

Tab. 2 – 6 – 1 Part data of potentiometric titration

V/mL	E/mV	$\Delta E/\text{mV}$	$\Delta V/\text{mL}$	$\Delta E/\Delta V$ /(mV/mL)	$\bar{V}/\text{mL}$	$\Delta^2 E$	$\Delta(\Delta E/\Delta V)$	$\Delta^2 E/\Delta V^2$
......	......							
10.00	168							
		34	1.00	34	10.50			
11.00	202						—	
		16	0.20	80	11.10			
11.20	218							
		7	0.05	140	11.225			
11.25	225($E1$)						120	2 400
		13(ΔE_1)	0.05	260	11.275			
11.30	238($E2$)						280	5 600
		27(ΔE_2)	0.05	540	11.325	14($\Delta^2 E_1$)		
11.35	265($E3$)						−20	−400
		26(ΔE_3)	0.05	520	11.375	−1($\Delta^2 E_2$)		
11.40	291($E4$)						−220	4 400
		15	0.05	300	11.425			
11.45	306							
		10	0.05	200	11.475		—	
11.50	316							
......	......							

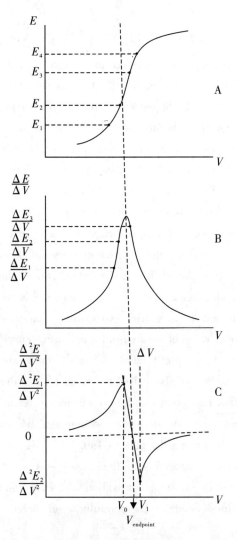

Fig. 2 – 6 – 2 Titration data processing curve of 0. 1 mol/l AgNO$_3$
solution titrating sodium chloride solution

Seeing from Fig. 2 – 6 – 2, if $\triangle V$ is small enough and equal, $\dfrac{\Delta^2 E}{\Delta V^2} \rightarrow \dfrac{\mathrm{d}^2 E}{\mathrm{d} V^2}$, the curve segment near the titration end point can be approximately regarded as a straight line, so the end point of the secondary micro-commercial law according to the similar triangles principle is:

$$\left| \frac{\Delta^2 E_1}{\Delta V^2} \right| \bigg/ \frac{\Delta E_2}{\Delta V^2} = \frac{V_{\text{endpoint}} - V_0}{V_1 - V_{\text{endpoint}}} \Rightarrow V_{\text{endpoint}} = \frac{\mid \Delta^2 E_1 \mid V_1 + \mid \Delta^2 E_2 \mid V_0}{= \mid \Delta^2 E_1 \mid + \mid \Delta^2 E_2 \mid},$$

Due to $V_1 = V_0 + \Delta V$, $\Delta E_1 = E_2 - E_1$, $\Delta E_2 = E_3 - E_2$, $\Delta E_3 = E_4 - E_3$, $\Delta^2 E_1 = \Delta E_2 - \Delta E_1 = E_3 - 2E_2 + E_1$, $\Delta^2 E_2 = E_4 - 2E_3 + E_2$, so:

$$V_{endpoint} = V_0 + \frac{\mid E_3 - 2E_2 + E_1 \mid \cdot \Delta V}{\mid E_3 - 2E_2 + E_1 \mid + \mid E_4 - 2E_3 + E_2 \mid}$$

Generally speaking, the three methods are used to determine the end point as follows: ① $E - V$ curve method. Take the titration volume (V) as the abscissa and the potentiometer read as the ordinate to draw an S-shaped curve, it is shown in Fig. 2 – 6 – 2A. The turning point(breaking point) of the curve is the end point of the the titration, which is convenient, but it is required that the potential jump at chemical measurement point of the titration is obvious. ② $\Delta E/\Delta V - V$ curve method. The data $\Delta E/\Delta V$ in Tab. 2 – 6 – 1 to the average volume(when calculating ΔE value, the volume of the average value between the front volume and the back volume) is plotted to obtain a curve, as shown in Fig. 2 – 6 – 2B. The volume corresponding to the highest point of the peak curve is the volume of the titration end point. The abscissa of the point coincides with the abscissa of the inflection point of the $\Delta E/\Delta V - V$ curve, as shown by the vertical dotted line in the figure. This method is also called the first-order micro quotient method. ③ $\Delta^2 E/\Delta V^2 - V$ curve method. Plot volume (V) with data $\Delta^2 E/\Delta V^2$ in Tab. 2 – 6 – 1 to get a curve with two extreme values, as shown in Fig. 2 – 6 – 2C. Generally, the maximum value of the first-order derivative curve is the end point, then the second-order derivative must be equal to zero, and this point is also the end point, as shown in Fig. 2 – 6 – 2C. This method is also called the second-order derivative method. Since the curve line near the titration end point can be approximately regarded as a straight line, the end point of the two-stage micro quotient method can also be determined by interpolation instead of the drawing method using the data in Tab. 2 – 6 – 1.

Seeing from the above, compared with the known end point calculation method, this method has the characteristics of simple derivation and easy calculation, and the result is accurate. Only a few values need to be carefully read before and after the chemical calculation point.

Sodium glycerophosphate is a mixture of α-glycerophosphate disodium salt pentahydrate and β-glycerophosphate disodium salt pentahydrate, contains not less than 98.0% percent and not more than 102.0% of $C_3H_7Na_2O_6P$, calculated on the anhydrous basis.

The structure of sodium glycerophosphate is as Fig. 2 – 6 – 3.

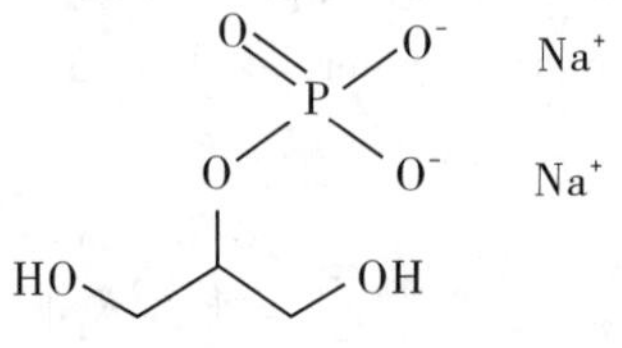

Fig. 2 – 6 – 3 Chemical structure of sodium glycerophosphate

Molecular formula is $C_3H_7Na_2O_6P \cdot 5H_2O$. Molecular weight is 306.11. Molecular weight without water is 216. 11. Assay reaction is as follows:

$$2\ C_3H_7Na_2O_6P + H_2SO_4 = 2\ C_3H_7NaHO_6P\ +\ Na_2SO_4$$

Molar ratio is 2 : 1. 1 mL of sulphate acid VS (0. 05 mol/L) is equivalent to 21. 66 mg of $C_3H_7Na_2O_6P$.

3 Instruments and Reagents

3. 1 Instruments

Analytical balance, potentiometric titrator, 10 mL burette, glass electrode, calomel electrode.

3. 2 Reagents

Sulfuric acid VS (0. 05 mol/L), phenolphthalein indicator, sodium glycerophosphate.

4 Experimental Procedures

Dissolve about 0. 2 g of sodium glycerophosphate, accurately weighed, in 30 mL of water, add 4 drops of phenolphthalein indicator solution, titrate with sulfuric acid VS(0. 05 mol/L) until the solution becomes colorless. According to potentiometric titration (General Rule 0701), titrate with sulfuric acid VS (0. 05 mol/L). 1 mL of sulfuric acid VS(0. 05 mol/L) is equivalent to 21. 6 mg of $C_5H_7N_2O_6P$.

At the same time during the titration, the glass electrode and the calomel electrode are inserted into the titration solution and connected to the potentiometric titration device. Record the potential value after adding different volumes of titration solution. In addition, when the titration is near the end point, record the potential value when each 0. 10 mL of the titration solution is added. The volume of the titration solution required at the end point is calculated with the first-order derivative or second-order derivative method, and the content is calculated.

5 Precautions

(1) The speed of electromagnetic stirring should not be too fast during the titration, and it is better not to produce air vortex.

(2) The volume and potential of the titrant should be recorded accurately.

(3) The interval of titration volume should not be too large, it can be carried out by 1 drop(0. 05 mL).

(4) The content can be estimated first, and the titrant can be added in the same volume near the end point[98% × molecular weight($C_5H_7N_2O_6P$)/molecular weight($C_3H_7Na_2O_6P \cdot 5H_2O$) = 98% ×216. 11/306. 11 =69. 19%].

6 Questions

(1) What are the characteristics of potentiometric titration?

(2) How to reduce the error of potential measurement?

(3) Why is the test solution titrated with sulfuric acid until phenolphthalein is colorless

before the content of sodium glycerophosphate is determined by potentiometric determination?

（4）Compare the advantages and disadvantages for indicator method and potential method.

References

［1］ Chinese Pharmacopoeia Commission. Chinese pharmacopoeia （2020 edition, Part Ⅱ） ［M］. Beijing: China Medical Science Press, 2020: 349.

［2］ XU X J. A simple method for calculating the end point of potentiometric titration ［J］. Guangdong pharmacy, 1997 （3）: 25 – 26.

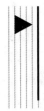

实验七　高效液相色谱法测定头孢氨苄胶囊含量

一、目的要求

（1）学习高效液相色谱分析的原理。

（2）学习外标法测定组分含量的方法。

（3）了解高效液相色谱仪的结构及正确使用方法。

（4）了解内标法、外标法、归一化法计算含量的应用范围及优缺点。

二、实验原理

以液体为流动相的色谱法称为液相色谱法。高效液相色谱法是用高压输液泵将具有不同极性的单一溶剂或不同比例的混合溶剂、缓冲液等流动相泵入装有固定相的色谱柱，经进样阀注入供试液，由流动相带入柱内，在柱内依据不同原理分离后，各成分先后进入检测器，色谱信号由记录仪或积分仪记录，从而达到分离分析的目的（图2－7－1）。该方法已成为化学、药学、医学、工业、农学、商检和法检等学科领域中重要的分离分析技术。

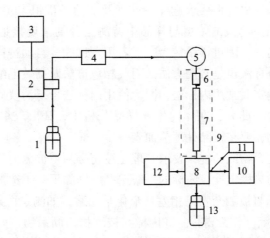

高效液相色谱流程：溶剂贮器（1）中的流动相被泵（2）吸入，经梯度控制器（3）按一定的梯度进行混合后输出，经压力控制器（4）测其压力和流量，导入进样阀（器）（5）经保护柱（6）、分离柱（7）后到检测器（8）检测（9 为柱温箱），由数据处理设备（10）处理数据或记录仪（11）记录色谱图，馏分收集器（12）收集馏分，最后进入废液瓶（13）收集废液。

图2－7－1　高效液相色谱流程

　　高效液相色谱法不需要样品气化，不受样品挥发性的约束，对于挥发性低、热稳定性差、分子量大的高分子化合物及离子性化合物尤其有利，可被用于氨基酸、蛋白质、核酸、生物碱、类脂、甾体、维生素、抗生素等分析。分子量较大，沸点较高的药物及无机盐类也可用高效液相色谱法进行分析。

　　高效液相色谱法的定量常采用外标法和内标法。外标法又称校正法或定量进样法，以供试品的对照品作为参照物质，相对比较以求得供试品的含量。外标法又分为工作曲线法和外标一点法。

　　工作曲线法就是用待测组分的对照品配制一系列不同浓度 $[(C_i)_{RS}]$ 的对照品溶液（至少 5 个浓度，不包括 0 点），准确进样，测量峰面积 $(A_i)_{RS}$ 或峰高 $(h_i)_{RS}$（相邻两峰未能基线分离时），与 $(C_i)_{RS}$ 绘制峰面积与浓度的标准曲线，然后在相同条件下，注入同量样品溶液，测量待测组分的峰面积，根据标准曲线，计算样品中待测组分的浓度。

　　外标一点法就是用一种浓度的 i 组分的对照品溶液对比测定样品溶液中 i 组分含量的方法。对照品溶液在相同条件下多次进样，所得峰面积的平均值用下式计算含量：

$$C_i = A_i \cdot (C_i)_{RS} / (A_i)_{RS},$$

式中，C_i 与 A_i 分别代表样品中 i 组分的浓度及相应的面积，$(C_i)_{RS}$ 与 $(A_i)_{RS}$ 代表对照品溶液中 i 组分浓度及相应面积。

　　内标法是指将一个样品中不含有的、已知质量的纯物质加入待测样品溶液中，以此纯物质的量为参比，对比测定 i 组分含量的方法。

　　外标一点法方法简单，但要求进样量准确及实验条件恒定，为了降低实验误差，应尽量使配制的对照品溶液的浓度与样品中待测组分的浓度接近，进样体积最好相等。在高效液相色谱中，因进样量较大，或者用六通阀、自动进样器进样，进样量误差相对较小，因此外标法也是常用方法。而气相色谱法及高效毛细电泳因进样量体积小，误差大，定量测定时常用内标法，因为使用内标法可抵消仪器稳定性差、进样量不准确等带来的误差。此外，在体内生物样品分析中，HPLC 法及 HPLC-MS 法也常采用内标法，内标物需要在样品处理前加入。

　　供选作内标的化合物或药物，要求其理化性质必须与被测物质十分相近，内标与被测组分具有相同的热稳定性，内标的一般选择原则如下：①选被测药物的同位素标记物为内标。②内标与被测药物只相差一个化学元素，如测定血浆中 5 - 氟尿嘧啶含量时，可用 5 - 氯尿嘧啶作为内标。③内标与被测物为同系物，如顶空气相色谱法测定血中乙醇浓度时，可用丙醇作为内标。④内标与被测物结构相似，如测定血中苯巴比妥为浓度时，选择去氧巴比妥作为内标。⑤选择结构不相似的化合物作内标，但其理化性质应与被测药物相近，如测定血浆中咖啡因的含量，可用卡马西平作为内标。

三、实验仪器与试剂

（一）仪器

高效液相色谱仪、分析天平、超声清洗仪、100 mL 量瓶、50 mL 量瓶、5 mL 移液管。

（二）试剂

头孢氨苄胶囊、甲醇、3.86% 醋酸钠溶液、4% 醋酸溶液、水。

四、实验方法

色谱仪：高效液相色谱仪；色谱柱：ODS 柱（4.6 mm×250 mm，5 μm）；柱温：室温；流动相：水－甲醇－3.86% 醋酸钠溶液－4% 醋酸溶液（742：240：15：3）；检测波长：254 nm。

五、含量测定

照高效液相色谱法［《中国药典》（2020 年版）通则 0512］测定。

供试品溶液：取头孢氨苄胶囊 20 粒，分别精密称重后，取开囊帽，倾出内容物，用小毛刷或其他适宜器具将囊壳内外拭净，并依次称重每一囊壳，用毛重减去囊壳质量，求出每粒内容物的装量和平均装量。

将每粒装量分别与平均装量相比较，计算出该粒装量差异的百分率。根据胶囊剂装量差异限度的规定，判定该批头孢氨苄胶囊装量差异是否符合规定。

取装量差异项下的内容物，倾入一乳钵中，用杵研磨，混合均匀，精密称取适量（约相当于头孢氨苄 0.1 g），置 100 mL 量瓶中，加流动相适量，充分振摇，使头孢氨苄溶解，再加流动相稀释至刻度，摇匀，滤过，精密量取续滤液 10 mL，置 50 mL 量瓶中，用流动相稀释至刻度，摇匀，用 0.45 μm 微孔滤膜过滤。

对照品溶液：取头孢氨苄对照品适量，精密称定，加流动相溶解并定量稀释制成每毫升中约含头孢氨苄（按 $C_{14}H_{17}N_2O_4S$）0.2 mg 的溶液。

系统适用性溶液：取供试品溶液适量，在 80 ℃ 水浴中加热 60 min，冷却。

色谱条件：用十八烷基硅烷键合硅胶为填充剂，以水－甲醇－3.86% 醋酸钠溶液－4% 醋酸溶液（742：240：15：3）为流动相；检测波长为 254 nm；系统适用性溶液进样体积为 20 μL，其他溶液进样体积为 10 μL。

系统适用性要求：系统适用性溶液色谱图中，头孢氨苄峰与相邻杂质峰之间的分离度应符合要求。

测定法：精密量取供试品溶液与对照品溶液，分别注入液相色谱仪，记录色谱图。按外标法以峰面积计算供试品中 $C_{14}H_{17}N_2O_4S$ 的含量。

六、注意事项

（1）流动相必须预先脱气，可用超声波、机械真空泵或水力抽气泵脱气。

（2）将配好的流动相接到流路中，开启泵起动开关，检测是否漏液。

（3）严格防止气泡进入系统，吸液软管必须充满流动相，吸液管的烧结不锈钢过滤器必须始终浸在溶剂中，若变换溶剂，必须先停泵，再将过滤器移到新的溶剂瓶内，然后才能开泵使用。

（4）溶剂的变换必须注意溶剂的极性和互溶性。当交换的溶剂与原溶剂能互溶时，从一种溶剂变换为另一种溶剂可通过直接用变换的溶剂彻底冲洗管路系统来实现；当交换的溶剂与原溶剂不能互溶时，必须注意他们的极性，要选择一种或两种溶剂都能互溶的溶剂（过渡溶剂）来冲洗管路系统，然后再用变换的溶剂来冲洗管路系统，才能实现溶剂的变换。

七、预习提要

（1）内标法与外标法的原理、方法及特点。

（2）怎样选择流动相？流动相中水的作用是什么？

（3）内标物应具备哪些条件？

八、思考题

（1）由于操作不当，系统中混入了气泡，对测定有何影响？如何排除这些气泡？

（2）变换溶剂时，直接将一种互不相溶的溶剂替换前一种溶剂时，对色谱行为有何影响？

参考文献

[1] 国家药典委员会. 中华人民共和国药典（2020 年版二部）［M］.北京：中国医药科技出版社，2020：349.

[2] 徐新军，谭奥，徐明辉. 内标法在液相色谱应用中的局限性［J］.中国药事，1998（6）：68－69.

Experiment 7 Assay of Cephalexin Capsules by HPLC

1 Purposes

(1) To learn the principle of HPLC analysis.

(2) To learn the method of external standard to determine the content of components.

(3) To understand the structure and proper use of HPLC.

(4) To understand the application range, advantages and disadvantages of internal standard method, external standard method and normalization method for content calculation.

2 Principles

The chromatographic method with liquid as mobile phase is called liquid chromatography. HPLC method is to use high pressure infusion pump to pump a single solvent, mixed solvent or buffer with different polarity and different proportion as mobile phase into a stationary phase chromatographic column. After the sample is injected through the injection valve, it is brought into the column by the mobile phase. After the compounds are separated according to different principles, each component enters the detector successively, and the chromatographic signal is recorded by the recorder or integrator, to achieve the purpose of separation and analysis(Fig. 2 – 7 – 1). This method has become an important separation and analysis technology in the fields of chemistry, pharmacy, medicine, industry, agriculture, commodity inspection and forensic identification.

HPLC does not require sample gasification and is not constrained by sample volatility. It is especially favorable for high molecular and ionic compounds with low volatility, poor thermal stability and high molecular weight. It can be used for the analysis of amino acids, proteins, nucleic acids, alkaloids, lipids, steroids, vitamins and antibiotics. High performance liquid chromatography can also be used for the analysis of drugs and inorganic salts with high molecular weight and high boiling point.

External standard method and internal standard method are often used for quantitative analysis of HPLC. External standard method, also known as calibration method or quantitative injection method, takes the reference substance of the test sample as the reference material, and obtains the content of the test sample by relative comparison. It can be divided into working curve method and external standard one point method.

The working curve method is to prepare a series of reference solutions$[(C_i)_{RS}]$ (at least 5 concentrations, excluding 0 point) with the reference substance of the components to be tested, and accurately inject samples, and measure the peak area$[(A_i)_{RS}]$ or peak height $[(h_i)_{RS}]$, (when the two adjacent peaks can not be separated by baseline), the working curve

127

is drawn with(C_i)$_{RS}$ method, and the content of sample solution is calculated by using this curve or its regression equation. The peak area (or peak height) is measured by the instrument, and the standard curve of peak area and concentration is made. Then, under the same conditions, the same amount of sample solution is injected to measure the peak area of the component to be measured, and the concentration of the component to be measured in the sample is calculated according to the standard curve.

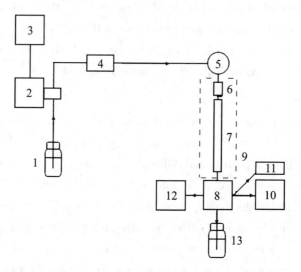

The procedure for the high performance liquid chromatography is as follows: the mobile phase in the solvent bottle(1) is inhaled by a pump(2) and is mixed in gradient controller(3) according to certain gradient and then output. The pressure and flow are measured by a pressure sensor(4). The samples are loaded on the flow path through injection valve(5) and flow through the protection column(6), the separation column(7) and then to the detector(8). The data is processed by the data processing equipment (10) or to record chromatograph chart by a recorder(11). The fraction collector(12) is used to collect fraction. Finally, the waste liquid is collected by the waste tank(13).

Fig. 2 - 7 - 1　Technological process of HPLC

One point method of the external standard is a method to determine the content of component in the sample solution compared with a concentration of reference solution of component i. The reference solution is injected many times under the same condition. The average value of the peak area is calculated by the following formula:

$$C_i = A_i \cdot (C_i)_{RS} / (A_i)_{RS}$$

where C_i and A_i represent the concentration and corresponding area of component i in the sample respectively, $(C_i)_{RS}$ and $(A_i)_{RS}$ represent the concentration and corresponding area of component i in the reference solution.

Internal standard method refers to the method of comparing and determining the content of component i by adding a known weight of pure substance which is not contained in a sample into the solution of the sample to be tested.

One point method of the external standard is simple, but it requires accurate injection volume and constant experimental conditions. In order to reduce the experimental error, the concentration of the prepared reference solution should be close to the concentration of the components to be measured in the sample, and the injection volume should be the same. In HPLC, the error of injection volume is relatively small due to the large injection volume or the use of six-way valve and automatic injector, so the external standard method is also commonly used. However, the internal standard method is commonly used in the quantitative determination of gas chromatography and high-performance capillary electrophoresis because the internal standard method can offset the poor stability of the instrument and the inaccurate injection volume error. In addition, the internal standard method is often used in HPLC and HPLC-MS methods for biological sample analysis, and the internal standard should be added before sample pretreatment.

The physical and chemical properties of the compounds or drugs to be used as internal standards must be very similar to those of the substances to be tested, and the internal standards and the components to be tested have the same thermal stability. The basic principles on how to choose an internal standard are as follows: ①The isotope markers of the drugs to be tested are selected as internal standards. ②There is only one chemical element difference between the internal standards and the drugs to be tested. For example, 5-fluorouracil can be used in the determination of 5-fluorouracil in plasma, the internal standard is 5-chlorouracil. ③ The internal standard is homologous with the tested substance, for example, propanol can be used as the internal standard when determining the concentration of ethanol in blood by headspace gas chromatography. ④The internal standard is similar to the tested substance in structure, for example, when determine the concentration of phenobarbital in blood, deoxybarbital is selected as the internal standard. ⑤ Compounds with different structures are selected as the internal standard, but their physical and chemical properties should be similar to the tested drug. For the determination of caffeine in plasma, carbamazepine can be used as internal standard.

3 Instruments and Reagents

3.1 Instruments

High performance liquid chromatography, analytical balance, ultrasonic cleaning instrument, 100 mL volumetric flask, 50 mL volumetric flask, 5 mL pipette.

3.2 Reagents

Cephalexin capsules, methanol, 3.86% sodium acetate solution, 4% acetic acid solution, water.

4 Experimental Method

Chromatograph: Shimadzu high performance liquid chromatograph; chromatographic column: ODS column(4. 6 mm × 250 mm, 5 μm); column temperature: room temperature; mobile phase: water-methanol- 3. 86% sodium acetate solution- 4% acetic acid solution (742 : 240 : 15 : 3); detection wavelength: 254 nm.

5 Content Determination

Determination by high performance liquid chromatography(General Rule 0512).

Test solution: Take 20 capsules of cefalexin, weigh each capsule accurately, open each capsule without loss of shell material, take off the capsule cap, pour out the contents, wipe the inside and outside of the capsule shell with a small brush or other suitable tools, weigh the shell of each capsule in turn, and calculate the net weight of each capsule by subtracting the weight shell from the respective gross weight.

Compare the each weight with the average weight, calculate the percentage of the weight variation and judge if it meets the requirement for the test of weight variation.

Mix the powder in the mortar using a pestle, and transfer an accurately weighted quantity of the freshing mixted powder, equivalent to about 0. 1 g of cefalexin, to a 100 mL volumetric flask. Add suitable amount of mobile phase, shaking well till cefalexin dissolved. Dilute with mobile phase to volume, mix and filter. Accurately measure 10 mL of the secondary filtrate and put it into a 50 mL volumetric flask. Dilute to volume with mobile phase, mix and filter through 0. 45 μm membrane filter.

Reference solution: Take an appropriate amount of cefalexin reference substance, weigh it precisely, add mobile phase to dissolve and dilute it to make a solution containing about 0. 2 mg of Cefalexin(as $C_{14}H_{17}N_2O_4S$) per mL.

System suitability solution: Taking an appropriate amount of cefalexin test solution, heat it at 80 ℃ water bath for 60 min, and then cool it.

The chromatographic conditions: Use octadecyl silane bonded silica gel as the filler, and water-methanol- 3. 86% sodium acetate solution- 4% acetic acid solution(742 : 240 : 15 : 3) as the mobile phase. The detection wavelength is 254 nm; the injection volume of system suitability solution is 20 μL, and the injection volume of other solutions are 10 μL.

The requirements for system suitability: The system suitability requires that the resolution between the cephalexin peak and the adjacent impurity peak in the chromatogram of the system applicability solution should meet the requirements.

Assay: Separately inject equal volumes(about 10 μL) of the standard solution and a filtered aliquot of the solution under test into the chromatograph, record the chromatograms and measure the responses for the major peaks. Calculate the percentage of $C_{14}H_{17}N_2O_4S$ in the test substances by the peak area by the external standard method.

6　Precautions

(1) The mobile phase must be degassed in advance and can be degassed by ultrasonic, mechanical vacuum or hydraulic pump.

(2) Connect the prepared mobile phase to the flow path. Open the pump start switch and detect whether there is liquid leakage.

(3) Strictly prevent air bubbles from entering the system, the suction hose must be filled with mobile phase. The sintered stainless-steel filter of the suction hose must always be immersed in the solvent. If the solvent is changed, the pump must be stopped first, and then the filter is moved to the new solvent bottle before the pump can be turned on.

(4) The change of solvent must be paid attention to the polarity and mutual solubility of solvent. When the transformed solvents and the original are miscible, the conversion from one solvent to another can be realized directly by thoroughly flushing the pipeline system with the transformed solvent. When the transformed solvents and the original can't be miscible, then must pay attention to their polarities. Under this circumstance, it is necessary to select one or two solvents that can dissolve each other(transition solvent) to flush the pipeline system, and then use the transformed solvent to flush the pipeline system, so that the transformation of the solvent can be realized.

7　Previews

(1) To master the principles, methods and characteristics of internal and external standard methods.

(2) How to choose mobile phase? What is the role of water in a mobile phase?

(3) What are the requirements for internal standards?

8　Questions

(1) Due to improper operation, air bubbles are mixed into the system. What are the effects of measurement? How do you get rid of these bubbles?

(2) What is the effect on the chromatogram behavior when a solvent is replaced directly by a non-dissolving solvent?

References

[1] Chinese Pharmacopoeia Commission. Chinese pharmacopoeia (2020 edition, Part Ⅱ) [M]. Beijing: China Medical Science Press, 2020: 349.

[2] XU X J, TAN A, XU M H. Limitations of internal standard method in liquid chromatography [J]. Chinese pharmaceutical affairs, 1998 (6): 68 – 69.

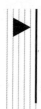

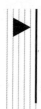

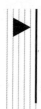

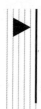

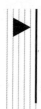

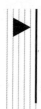

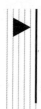

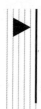

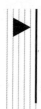

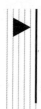

实验八　气相色谱法测定维生素 E 软胶囊含量

一、实验目的

（1）掌握气相色谱法分析的原理。
（2）学习气相色谱仪的一般操作技术及其使用要点。
（3）掌握气相色谱法测定维生素 E 软胶囊含量的原理和方法。

二、实验原理

气相色谱仪是用于分离复杂样品中的化合物的化学分析仪器。气相色谱仪中有一根流通型的狭长管道，这就是色谱柱。在色谱柱中，不同的样品因为具有不同的物理和化学性质，与特定的柱填充物（固定相）有着不同的相互作用而被流动相（载气）以不同的速率带动。当化合物从柱的末端流出时，被检测器检测到，产生相应的信号，并被转化为电信号输出。检测器用于检测柱的流出物，从而确定每一个组分到达色谱柱末端的时间及每一个组分的含量。通常来说，人们通过物质流出柱（被洗脱）的顺序和它们在柱中的保留时间来表征不同的物质。影响物质流出柱的顺序及保留时间的因素包括载气的流速、温度等。

常见气相色谱仪装置见图 2 - 8 - 1。

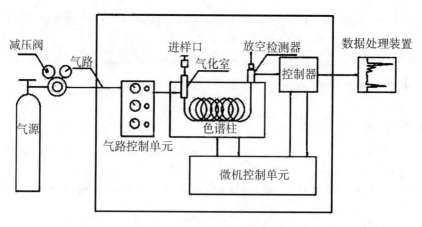

图 2 - 8 - 1　气相色谱仪结构

维生素 E（vitamin E）有合成型和天然型两类；合成型维生素 E 为（±）- 2,

132

5，7，8－四甲基－2－（4，8，12－三甲基十三烷基）－6－苯并二氢吡喃醇醋酸酯或 dl-α-生育酚醋酸酯，天然型维生素 E 为（+）－2，5，7，8－四甲基－2－（4，8，12－三甲基十三烷基）－6－苯并二氢吡喃醇醋酸酯或 d-α-生育酚醋酸酯。其结构见图 2-8-2。

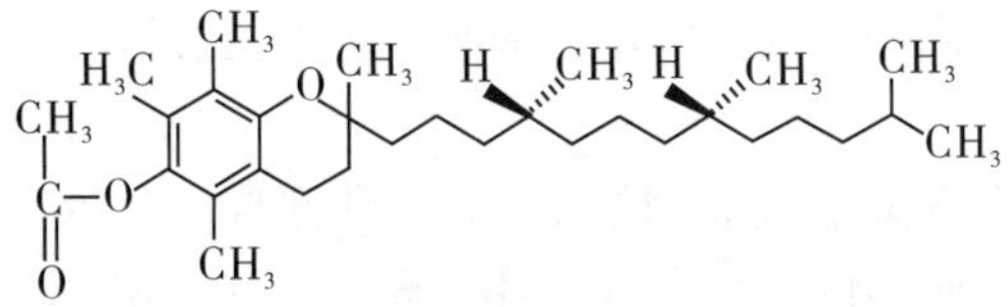

图 2-8-2 维生素 E 的化学结构

维生素 E 是一种脂溶性维生素，其水解产物为生育酚，是最主要的抗氧化剂之一。维生素 E 溶于脂肪和乙醇等有机溶剂中，不溶于水，对热、酸稳定，对碱不稳定，对氧敏感，对热不敏感，但油炸时维生素 E 活性明显降低。

气相色谱法是集分离与测定于一体的分析方法，适合于多组分混合物的定性定量分析。该法具有高度选择性，可分离维生素 E 及其异构体，选择性地测定维生素 E，目前该法为各国药典所采用。尽管维生素 E 的沸点高达 350 ℃，但仍可无须衍生化直接用气相色谱法测定含量，测定时均采用内标法，内标的选择原则见实验七。

三、实验仪器与试剂

（一）仪器
气相色谱仪、水浴锅、棕色具塞锥形瓶、HP-1 毛细管柱。

（二）试剂
维生素 E 对照品、维生素 E 软胶囊、无水乙醇、硝酸、正三十二烷、正己烷。

四、实验步骤

（一）鉴别
（1）取本品内容物适量（约相当于维生素 E 30 mg），加无水乙醇 10 mL 溶解后，加硝酸 2 mL，摇匀，在 75 ℃加热约 15 min，观察并记录实验现象（溶液应显橙红色）。

（2）在含量测定项下记录的色谱图中，供试品溶液主峰的保留时间应与对照品溶液主峰的保留时间一致。

（二）含量测定
照气相色谱法［《中国药典》（2020 年版）通则 0521］测定。

色谱条件与系统适用性试验：以硅酮（OV-17）为固定相，涂布浓度为 2%；或

133

以 HP-1 毛细管柱（100%二甲基聚硅氧烷）为分析柱，柱温为 265 ℃。理论板数按维生素 E 峰计算应不低于 500（填充柱）或 5 000（毛细管柱），维生素 E 峰与内标物质峰的分离度应大于 2。

校正因子测定：取正三十二烷适量，加正己烷溶解并稀释成每毫升中含 1.0 mg 的溶液，摇匀，作为内标溶液。另取维生素 E 对照品约 20 mg，精密称定，置棕色具塞锥形瓶中，精密加入内标溶液 10 mL，密塞，振摇使溶解；取 1～3 μL 注入气相色谱仪，计算校正因子。

测定法：取维生素 E 软胶囊 20 粒，分别精密称重后，依次放置于固定位置，用剪刀或刀片划破囊壳，倾出内容物。囊壳用乙醚或乙醇等易挥发溶剂洗净，置通风处使溶剂自然挥干，持续大约 30 min，再依次精密称重每一囊壳，即可求出每粒内容物的装量和平均装量。

每粒内容物的质量之和除以 20 即得每粒平均装量，将每粒装量分别与平均装量相比较，计算出该粒装量差异的百分率，根据该规格胶囊装量差异限度的规定，判断维生素 E 软胶囊装量差异是否符合规定［《中国药典》（2020 年版）通则 0103］。

取装量差异项下的内容物，混合均匀，取适量（约相当于维生素 E 20 mg），精密称定，置棕色具塞锥形瓶中，精密加入内标溶液 10 mL，密塞，振摇使溶解；取 1～3 μL 注入气相色谱仪，测定，计算，即得。

五、注意事项

（1）实验用容器应干燥。
（2）供试品溶液与对照品溶液应避光保存。

六、思考题

（1）气相色谱法测定维生素 E 为什么采用内标法？
（2）试述气相色谱法的特点及分析适用范围。
（3）柱温能否超过柱内所涂固定液的最高使用温度，为什么？
（4）检测器温度必须高于柱温，为什么？

参考文献

国家药典委员会. 中华人民共和国药典（2020 年版二部）［M］. 北京：中国医药科技出版社，2020：1487.

Experiment 8　The Determination of Vitamin E Soft Capsules by Gas Chromatography

1　Purposes

(1) To master the principle of gas chromatography analysis.

(2) To learn the general operation technology of gas chromatograph and its practical points.

(3) To master the principle and method of the determination of vitamin E soft capsule by gas chromatography.

2　Principles

Gas chromatograph(GC) is a chemical analysis instrument used to separate compounds from complex samples. There is a long and narrow pipe in the gas chromatograph, which is the chromatographic column. In the chromatographic column, different samples are driven by gas flow(carrier gas, mobile phase) at different rates because of their different physical and chemical properties and different interactions with specific column fillers(stationary phase). When compounds flow from the end of the column, they are detected by the detector, generate the corresponding signal, and are converted into electrical signal output. The detector is used to detect the effluent of the column to determine the time at which each component reaches the end of the column and the content of each component. Generally speaking, different substances are characterized by the order in which substances flow out of the column(eluted) and their retention time in the column. The factors affecting the order and retention time of the material outflow column include the flow rate of carrier gas, temperature and so on.

Common gas chromatograph devices are shown in Fig. 2 – 8 – 1.

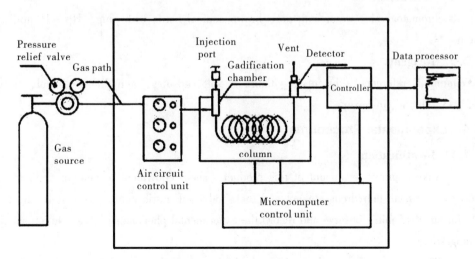

Fig. 2 – 8 – 1　Structure of gas chromatograph

Vitamin E is synthetic or natural. Synthetic vitamin E is(+)-2, 5, 7, 8-tetramethyl-2-(4, 8, 12-trimethyl tridecyl)-6-benzodihydropyranol acetic ester or *dl*-α-dimethyl-tocopherol acetate, natural vitamin E is (±)-2, 5, 7, 8-tetramethyl-2-(4, 8, 12-trimethyltrialyl)-6-dihydropyranol acetate, or *d*-dimethyltocopherol acetate. The structure is shown in Fig. 2 − 8 − 2.

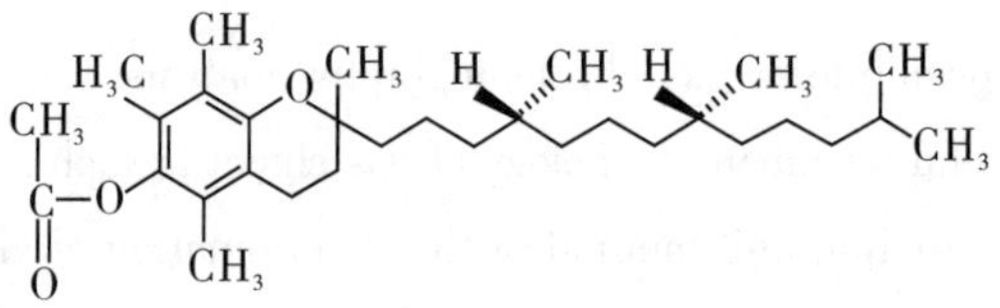

Fig. 2 − 8 − 2   Chemical structure of vitamin E

Vitamin E is a fat-soluble vitamin. Its hydrolyzed product is tocopherol, which is one of the most important antioxidants. Vitamin E is soluble in fat or organic solvents such as ethanol and insoluble in water. It's stable to heat and acid and unstable to alkali, sensitive to oxygen and insensitive to heat. But the activity of vitamin E is significantly reduced in frying.

Gas chromatography is a method of separation and determination which is suitable for qualitative and quantitative analysis of multicomponent mixtures. The method is highly selective, which can separate vitamin E and its isomers and is used to determine vitamin E selectively. At present, this method is adopted by various national pharmacopoeia. Although vitamin E's boiling point is 350 ℃, it can be determined by GC directly without derivation. The content determination is using internal standard method. The selection principle of internal standard is shown in Experiment 7.

3   Instruments and Reagents

3.1   Instruments

Gas chromatograph, water bath pot, brown conical bottle with plug, Hp − 1 capillary column.

3.2   Reagents

Vitamin E reference substance, vitamin E soft capsules, anhydrous ethanol, nitric acid, n-32 alkane, n-hexane.

4   Experimental Procedures

4.1   Identification

(1) Take appropriate amount of this product (about equivalent to vitamin E 30 mg). Dissolve it in 10 mL anhydrous ethanol and then add 2 mL nitric acid, shake well, heat at 75 ℃ for about 15 min, observe and record the experimental phenomena (the solution should be orange-red).

(2) The retention time of the main peak obtained from the test solution is identical with

that of the peak obtained from vitamin E reference substance.

4.2 Determination

Carry out the method for gas chromatography (General Rule 0521).

Chromatographic conditions and system suitability test: Use a column packed with 2% silicone (OV-17) as the stationary phase or HP-1 capillary column (100% dimethyl polysiloxane) as the analytical column and maintain the column temperature at 265 ℃. The number of theoretical plates of the column should be no less than 500 (packed column) or 5 000 (capillary column), calculated with reference to the peak of vitamin E, and the resolution factor between the peaks of vitamin E and internal standard is not less than 2.

Calibration factor determination: Dissolve a quantity of n-32 alkane in n-hexane to produce a solution of 1.0 mg per mL as the internal standard solution. Accurately weigh 20 mg of vitamin E reference substance and put it in a brown conical bottle with plug, accurately add 10 mL of internal standard solution, put it in the plug and shake it well; inject $1 \sim 3$ μL into the column and calculate the correction factor.

Assay: Weigh accurately 20 intact capsules individually to obtain their gross weights, taking care to preserve the identity of each capsule, then cut open the capsules with scissors or a sharp open blade, and remove the contents by washing with ethyl ether or ethanol. Allow the occluded solvent to evaporate from the shells at room temperature over a period of about 30 min. Weigh the individual shells, and calculate the net weight of content of each capsule.

The sum of the contents weight of each capsule is divided by 20 to get the average content of each capsule. Compare the content of each capsule with the average content respectively, calculate the percentage of the weight variation of the capsule, and judge whether the weight variation of vitamin E soft capsule meets the requirements (0103).

Take the contents under the weight variation, mix well, weigh accurately a propriate amount of the mixed contents equaling to 20 mg of vitamin E, put it in a brown conical bottle with plug, accurately add 10 mL of internal standard solution, put in the plug and shake well, inject $1 \sim 3$ μL into the column and calculate the content of vitamin E.

5 Precautions

(1) The containers for experiment should be dry.

(2) The test solution and reference solution should be kept away from light.

6 Questions

(1) Why use internal standard method for the determination of vitamin E by gas chromatography?

(2) Describe the features of gas chromatography and the scope of application for analysis.

(3) Can the column temperature exceed the highest usage temperature of the fixed

liquid applied in the column? Why?

(4) The temperature of detector must be higher than the column temperature. Why?

References

Chinese Pharmacopoeia Commission. Chinese pharmacopoeia (2020 edition, Part Ⅱ) [M]. Beijing: China Medical Science Press, 2020: 1487.

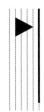

实验九 微流控芯片分析法测定赖氨酸颗粒剂中 赖氨酸的含量

一、目的要求

（1）学习微流控芯片分析法的原理。

（2）学习外标法测定主成分含量的方法。

（3）了解微流控芯片分析仪的结构与正确使用方法。

二、实验原理

微流控芯片（microfluidic chip），或称微全分析系统（micro total analysis system），是近年发展起来的一种新型的分离分析技术。它将进样、分离、检测，以及化学反应、药物筛选、细胞培养与分选等集成在几平方厘米的芯片上进行，具有高效、快速、微量、微型化等特点。目前的微流控芯片主要为芯片毛细管电泳，其原理是以高压电场为驱动力，以芯片毛细管为分离通道，依据样品中各组分之间淌度和分配行为等差异而实现高效、快速分离的一种电泳新技术。

简单的微流控芯片分析仪由高压电源、芯片和检测器组成。高压电源提供进样电压和分离电压。芯片设有进样通道和分离通道。电导检测器是较通用的检测器，适用于荷电成分的检测。本实验所用的非接触式电导检测器，其电极与溶液不接触，可避免电极污染中毒和高压干扰等问题，加上芯片与检测电极板之间相互独立，更换和清洗操作非常方便。

本实验采用外标法测定赖氨酸颗粒剂中赖氨酸的含量。外标法是以待测成分的对照品作为对照物，通过比较求得供试品的含量的方法。配制一系列浓度的标准液，在同一条件下测定，用峰面积（或峰高）与浓度制作标准曲线，然后在相同条件下，测定待测样品组分，根据标准曲线，计算样品中待测组分的浓度。

三、实验仪器与试剂

（一）仪器

微流控芯片分析仪（包括双路高压电源、非接触式电导检测器、十字通道芯片，均为中山大学药学院研制）、循环水式真空泵。

（二）试剂

L-赖氨酸对照品、0.2 mol/L 硝酸、0.1 mol/L NaOH、硼酸、乙二胺、超纯水、供试品 L-赖氨酸盐酸盐颗粒剂。

四、实验方法

（1）芯片的清洗：0.2 mol/L 硝酸清洗 5 min →超纯水清洗 5 min。

（2）芯片的活化：0.1 mol/L NaOH 活化 5 min →用超纯水清洗 5 min →用缓冲溶液（硼酸：乙二胺 =5 mmol/L：15 mmol/L）平衡 5 min。

测定：先在芯片储液池 a、c、e（图 2-9-1）中加入运行缓冲溶液（硼酸：乙二胺 = 5mmol/L：15 mmol/L），再向样品池 b 中加入供试品或对照品溶液。将高压电源的进样电源正负极分别置于储液池 b 和 c，分离电源正负极分别置于储液池 a 和 e。开启高压电源进入进样状态，在 b-c（进样通道）之间加进样电压 20 s（首次进样足够长时间，一般为 20～30 s，使样品达到 b-c 之间的分离通道 a-e），然后切换至分离电压 2.00 kV（可调）并同步启动数据工作站记录。重复进样 10 s，切换分离检测并记录。

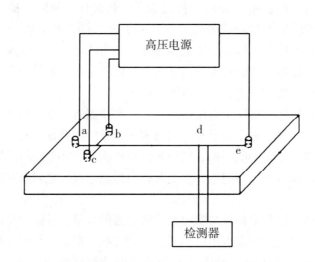

图 2-9-1 微流控芯片示意

五、含量测定

对照品的测定：取 L-赖氨酸对照品约 20 mg，精密称定至 10 mL 量瓶中，加超纯水溶解并稀释至刻度，摇匀，得浓度为 2.00 mg/mL 的对照品储备液。取 L-赖氨酸对照品储备液（2.00 mg/mL），配成浓度为 1.00×10^2 μg/mL、2.00×10^2 μg/mL、

$3.00 \times 10^2\, \mu g/mL$、$4.00 \times 10^2\, \mu g/mL$、$5.00 \times 10^2\, \mu g/mL$ 的系列标准溶液，在相同的实验条件下，分别进样，测量赖氨酸峰面积（或峰高），以峰面积（或峰高）对浓度做标准曲线。

样品的测定：取装量差异检查项下的赖氨酸颗粒剂适量（约相当于赖氨0.1 g），精密称定至 100 mL 量瓶中，用超纯水溶解，定容，摇匀，滤过，精密量取续滤液 2 mL，置 10 mL 量瓶中，用超纯水稀释至刻度，摇匀。在同对照品测定相同条件下进样，测量赖氨酸的峰面积，外标法计算含量。

六、结果处理

（1）标准曲线绘制。以所测量的系列标准溶液峰面积为纵坐标，浓度为横坐标，在 Excel 中绘制工作曲线：插入→图表→XY 散点图（选择平滑线散点图）→系列（添加）→取定 X 和 Y 所在的表格→得到标准曲线→右键选中曲线→添加趋势线→选项（勾选显示公式、显示 R^2 值），即得到回归方程。

（2）测得的样品溶液峰面积代入回归方程中，求得样品溶液的浓度，并计算样品中 L–赖氨酸的含量。

七、注意事项

（1）处理芯片时应每次用指定的溶液浸润 2 min 后，用真空泵抽动补液。活化与检测时务必保证通道无气泡（清洗活化过程中，从 1 个孔道真空抽气，同时保证另外 3 个孔道注满液体。加样时保证另外 3 个孔道注满缓冲溶液）。

（2）溶液均经 0.22 μm 的滤膜过滤。

（3）高压电源输出电流在安全范围，但仍须谨防身体接触高压电极。

（4）实验完毕要用水清洗通道，然后盖住芯片，以防灰尘侵入。

八、思考题

（1）比较高效液相色谱与微流控芯片测定药品含量的优缺点。

（2）为了改善微流控芯片测定药物含量的精密度，你认为可采用哪些措施？

实 验 报 告

年级：　　　　班：　　　　姓名：　　　　学号：

微流控芯片分析法测定赖氨酸颗粒剂中赖氨酸的含量

一、实验记录

仪器：微流控芯片分析仪型号_____编号：_____

分离电压：_____ kV　分离电流：_____ μA

进样时间：首次 20 s，重复进样 10 s

记录时长：_____ min

标准溶液或样品溶液	迁移时间	峰面积或峰高			
		第 1 次进样	第 2 次进样	第 3 次进样	平均值
1.00×10^2 μg/mL 赖氨酸					
2.00×10^2 μg/mL 赖氨酸					
4.00×10^2 μg/mL 赖氨酸					
6.00×10^2 μg/mL 赖氨酸					
8.00×10^2 μg/mL 赖氨酸					
10.00×10^2 μg/mL 赖氨酸					
赖氨酸盐酸盐颗粒剂					

二、数据处理与结果报告

1. 标准曲线

回归方程：　　　　　　　　　　　　　　相关系数：

2. 样品溶液的浓度（代入方程计算）

3. 赖氨酸盐酸盐颗粒剂中赖氨酸的含量

三、讨论

Experiment 9   Determination of Lysine in Lysine Granules by Microfluidic Chip Analysis

1   Purposes

(1) To learn the principle of microfluidic chip analysis.

(2) To learn the method of external standard to determine the content of principal components.

(3) To understand the structure and proper use of microfluidic chip analyzer.

2   Principles

Microfluidic chip, or micro total analysis system, is a new kind of separation analysis technology developed in recent years. It integrates sample injection, separation and detection, as well as chemical reaction, drug screening, cell culture and sorting on a few square centimeters chip. It is efficient, rapid, micro and microminiaturization. The current microfluidic chip, mainly chip capillary electrophoresis, is based on the high voltage electric field as the driving force, chip capillary as the separation channel and a new electrophoresis technology that achieves efficient and rapid separation according to the differences of mobility and distribution among the components in the sample.

The simple microfluidic chip analyzer is composed of high voltage power, chip and detector. The high voltage power provides the sampling voltage and separation voltage. The chip is equipped with injection channel and separation channel. Conductivity detector is a general detector, which is suitable for the detection of charged components. The non-contact conductivity detector used in this experiment, the electrode is not contact with the solution, which can avoid the problems of electrode contamination, poisoning and high-voltage interference. In addition, the chip is independent from the detection electrode plate, so it is very convenient to replace and clean.

The content of lysine in lysine granules is determined by external standard method. The external standard method is a method to compare the content of the tested product with the reference substance to be measured. A series of concentration of standard solutions are prepared, measured under the same conditions, and a standard curve is made with peak area (or peak height) against concentration. Then, the component of the sample under test is measured under the same conditions, and the concentration of the component under test is calculated according to the standard curve.

3   Instruments and Reagents

3. 1 Instruments

Microfluidic chip analyzer(including dual high-voltage power supply, non-contact conductivity detector and cross channel chip, all developed by school of pharmacy, Sun Yat-sen University), circulating water vacuum pump.

3. 2 Reagents

L-lysine reference substance, 0. 2 mol/L nitric acid, 0. 1 mol/L NaOH, boric acid, super pure water, ethylenediamine, sample is L-lysine hydrochloride granule.

4 Experimental Methods

(1) Chip cleaning: Use 0. 2 mol/L nitric acid to clean the chip for 5 min and high-purity water clean for 5 min.

(2) Activation of the chip: Use 0. 1 mol/L NaOH to activate the chip for 5 min, clean with high pure water for 5 min, and balance with buffer solution(boric acid: ethylenediamine = 5 mmol/L: 15 mmol/L) for 5 min.

Determination: First add the running buffer solution(boric acid: ethylenediamine = 5mmol/L : 15 mmol/L) into the chip reservoir a, c and e(as shown in Fig. 2 - 9 - 1), and then add the test or control solution to the sample pool b. The positive and negative electrodes of the incoming power source of the high-voltage power source are respectively placed in the reservoir b and c, and the positive and negative poles of the separated power source are respectively placed in the reservoir a and e. Turn on the high voltage power at the injection state, add the sample voltage of 20 s between b - c(the injection channel) (the first injection is long enough, generally 20 ~ 30 s, so that the sample reaches the separation channel a - e between b - c), then switch to the separation voltage of 2. 00 kV(adjustable) and start the data station record synchronously. Repeat sampling 10 s, switch to separate detection and record.

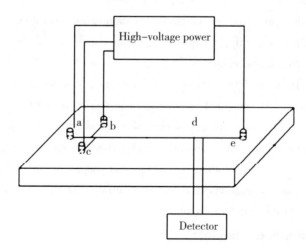

Fig. 2 - 9 - 1 Schematic diagram of microfluidic chip

5 Content Determination

Determination of reference substance: 20 mg of L-lysine reference substance is accurately weighed, and dissolve in high-purity water and its capacity is determined in a 10 mL volumetric flask. The reference stock solution with a concentration of 2.00 mg/mL is obtained. L-lysine reference stock solution(2.00 mg/mL) is prepared into a series of standard solutions with concentrations of 1.00×10^2 μg/mL, 2.00×10^2 μg/mL, 3.00×10^2 μg/mL, 4.00×10^2 μg/mL, and 5.00×10^2 μg/mL. Under the same experimental conditions, lysine peak area(or peak height) is measured and the standard curve of peak area(or peak height) and concentration is made.

Sample determination: The sample is accurately weighed(about 0.1 g of lysine) and dissolve in high pure water, with a capacity of 100 mL volumetric flask. The filtrate is shaken and filtered 2 mL of the secondary filtrate is accurately taken and put in 10 mL flask. The peak area of lysine is measured under the same condition.

6 Results Processing

(1) Draw standard curve by measuring a series of standard solution peak area as the ordinate, concentration as the abscissa, working curve is drawing in Excel: insert→charts→ *XY* scatterplot(choose smooth line scatterplot)→series(add)→*X* and *Y* in fixed form→get the standard curve→right-click the selected curve→add a trend line→options(check the display formula, R^2 value), the regression equation is obtained.

(2) The measured peak area of the sample solution is substituted into the regression equation to obtain the concentration of the sample solution and calculate the content of L-lysine in the sample.

7 Precautions

(1) The chip shall be soaked in the specified solution for 2 min each time, and the replenishment shall be drawn by vacuum pump. It is important to ensure that the channel is free of air bubbles during activation and detection(During cleaning and activation, vacuum the air from one channel and fill the other three channels with liquid. Make sure the other three channels are filled with the buffer solution when the sample is added).

(2) The solution is filtered with 0.22 μm filtration membrane.

(3) The output current of the high-voltage power supply is in the safe range, but it should be guarded against body contact with the high-voltage electrode.

(4) Clean the passage with water after the experiment, and then cover the chip to prevent the dust invasion.

8 Questions

(1) What are the advantages and disadvantages of high performance liquid

chromatography and microfluidic chip in the determination of drug content?

(2) In order to improve the precision of microfluidic chip in the determination of drug content, what measures can be taken?

Report

Grade: Class: Name: Student ID:

Determination of Lysine in Lysine Granules by Microfluidic Chip Analysis

1. Experimental Record

Instrument: microfluidic chip analyzer Type: _____ No: _____

Separation voltage: _____ kV   Separation current: _____ μA

Sampling time: 20 s for the first time, repeat sampling for 10 s

Recording duration: _____ min

Standard solution or sample solution	Migration time	Peak area or peak height			
		First injection	Second injection	Third injection	Average
1.00×10^2 μg/mL Lysine					
2.00×10^2 μg/mL Lysine					
4.00×10^2 μg/mL Lysine					
6.00×10^2 μg/mL Lysine					
8.00×10^2 μg/mL Lysine					
10.00×10^2 μg/mL Lysine					
Lysine hydrochloride granules					

2. Data Processing and Result Reporting

1. Standard curve

Regression equation: Correlation coefficient:

2. Concentration of sample solution(calculate by substituting equation)

3. Lysine content in lysine hydrochloride granules(calculation)

3. Discussion

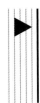 实验十　高效毛细管电泳分离检测苯磺酸氨氯地平对映异构体

一、目的要求

（1）学习高效毛细管电泳仪的原理。
（2）学习外标法测定主成分含量的方法。
（3）了解高效毛细管电泳仪的结构与正确使用方法。
（4）了解手性药物的分析方法。

二、实验原理

毛细管电泳（capillary electrophoresis，CE）又称为高效毛细管电泳（high performance capillary electrophoresis，HPCE），是一类以高压电场为驱动力，被分离组分在毛细管中按其淌度或分配系数不同进行高效、快速的分离，是在极细的毛细管内实现的一种新型液相微分离技术（图2-10-1）。

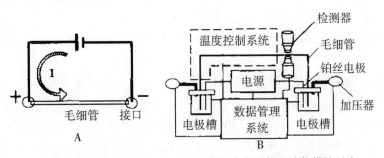

A.毛细管电泳电学原理示意；B.毛细管电泳实用装置功能模块示意

图2-10-1　毛细管电泳装置原理与结构

手性药物是指药物分子结构中引入手性中心后，得到的一对互为实物与镜像的对映异构体。这些对映异构体的理化性质基本相似，仅仅是旋光性有所差别，分别被命名为R-型（右旋）或S-型（左旋）、外消旋。一对对映异构体除旋光性外，在非手性环境中的物理化学性质几乎完全相同，但是，它们在手性环境下的表现是不同的。生命体系是一个手性环境，因此手性药物在生物体内的吸收、分布、代谢和排泄均体现出立体选择性，手性药物的不同对映异构体往往显示出不同的药理学和毒理学

特性及不同的药代动力学性质。本实验采用高效毛细管电泳仪分离检测苯磺酸氨氯地平片剂中对映异构体的含量。

外标法又称为校正法或定量进样法。本法要求能准确地定量进样，配置一系列浓度已知的对照品溶液，在同一操作条件下，按同量注入色谱仪，测量其峰面积（或峰高），作峰面积与浓度的标准曲线，然后在相同条件下，注入同量样品溶液，测量待测组分的峰面积（或峰高），根据标准曲线，计算样品中待测组分的浓度。采用外标法测定药物含量时，对照品溶液的浓度应与被测物浓度接近，以利于定量分析的准确性。

三、实验仪器与试剂

（一）仪器
高效毛细管电泳仪、石英毛细管柱（35 cm × 40 μm i.d.，有效长度 35 cm，河北永年光导纤维厂）。
（二）试剂
氨氯地平对照品、羟丙基 – β – 环糊精（HP-β-CD）、枸橼酸、三羟甲基氨基甲烷（Tris）、超纯水、氨氯地平片剂。

四、实验步骤

（1）配制 44 mmol/L 枸橼酸 + 30 mmol/L Tris + 35 mmol/L HP-β-CD 为电泳运行液。氨氯地平对照品配成 0.2 g/L 溶液备用。
（2）毛细管柱在使用前依次用 0.1 mol/L NaOH、超纯水和电泳运行液冲洗毛细管柱 5 min。
（3）分离电压 16 kV，压力进样 10 s。
（4）含量测定：取苯磺酸氨氯地平对照品适量，用超纯水配成浓度为 40 mg/L、80 mg/L、120 mg/L、160 mg/L、200 mg/L 的系列对照品溶液，分离电压 16 kV，压力进样 10 s，分别进样并记录色谱图。另取外消旋氨氯地平 1 片（标示含量为每片 5 mg）于 50 mL 容量瓶中，在适量水中用超声波辅助提取 10 min，定容，经过 0.45 μm 微孔滤膜过滤，同法测定。按外标法以峰面积计算供试品中苯磺酸氨氯地平的含量。

五、注意事项

（1）运行缓冲液应先超声脱气。
（2）缓冲液及样品须经过 0.45 μm 微孔滤膜过滤。
（3）仪器操作时一定要弹起电压启/停控制按钮，停止高压输出后（此时电压电流都显示0），才可以取出毛细管的进样端进样。

六、思考题

（1）什么是手性药物？手性药物有哪些特点？

（2）高效毛细管电泳的特点是什么？

（3）高效毛细管电泳有哪些分离模式？

（4）采用高效毛细管电泳拆分手性药物与采用高效液相色谱和气相色谱拆分手性药物各有何优势？

Experiment 10　High Performance Capillary Electrophoresis for Detection of Amlodipine Besylate Enantiomers

1　Purposes

(1) To learn the principle of high performance capillary electrophoresis meter.

(2) To learn the method of external standard to determine the content of principal components.

(3) To understand the structure and correct usage of high-performance capillary electrophoresis meter.

(4) To understand the analysis method for the chiral drugs.

2　Principles

Capillary electrophoresis(CE) , also known as high performance capillary electrophoresis (HPCE) , is a new kind of liquid phase micro separation technology, which is driven by high voltage electric field and separated by components in capillaries according to their mobility or distribution coefficients(Fig. 2 – 10 – 1) .

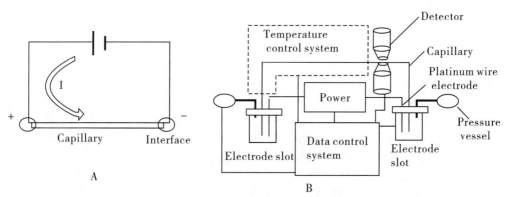

A.Electrical principle diagram;　B.Schematic diagram of functional module

Fig. 2 – 10 – 1　Principle and structure of capillary electrophoresis

Chiral drug refers to a pair of enantiomers that are physical and mirror images of each other due to the introduction of chiral center in the molecular structure of drugs. The physical and chemical properties of these enantiomers were basically similar, but the optical activity was different. They were named R-type (right-handed) or S-type (left-handed) and racemization respectively. Pairs of enantiomers have nearly identical physical and chemical properties in non-chiral environments except for optical rotation, but they behave differently in chiral environments. The life system is a chiral environment, so the absorption, distribution, metabolism and excretion of chiral drugs in the organism all reflect to the three-dimensional selectivity. Different enantiomers of chiral drugs often show different pharmacological and toxicological characteristics and different pharmacokinetic properties. The enantiomers of amlodipine benzenesulfonate tablets were determined by high performance capillary electrophoresis.

External standard method is also called correction method or quantitative sampling method. This method requires accurate quantitative injection, configures a series of known reference solutions and inject the same amount solutions into the chromatograph under the same operating conditions. Measuring the peak area (or peak height) and calculate the standard curve of peak area and concentration, and then under the same conditions, inject the same amount of sample solution, measure peak area(or peak height) of the component under test. According to the standard curve, calculate the concentration of the component under test in the sample. When the external standard method is used to determine the drug content, the concentration of the control solution should be close to the concentration of the substance to be measured, so as to facilitate the accuracy of quantitative analysis.

3　Instruments and Reagents

3.1 Instruments

Capillary electrophoresis meter, quartz capillary column(35 cm × 40 μm i. d. , effective length 35 cm, Hebei Yongnian Fiber Factory) .

3.2 Reagents

Amlodipine reference substance, HP-β-CD, citric acid, Tris, high-purity water, amlodipine tablet.

4　Procedures

(1) Prepare of 44 mmol/L citric acid + 30 mmol/L Tris + 35 mmol/L HP-β-CD as electrophoretic running liquid. Amlodipine control is prepared into 0. 2 g /L for use.

(2) The capillary column is rinsed with 0. 1 mol/L NaOH, ultra-pure water and electrophoresis running solution for 5 min.

(3) Separation voltage is 16 kV and pressure is 10 s.

(4) Determination: Appropriate amount of amlodipine benzenesulfonate control sample is taken, and the sample is prepared into a series of standard solutions with concentration of 40 mg/L, 80 mg/L, 120 mg/L, 160 mg/L, and 200 mg/L with ultra-pure water. The separation voltage is 16 kV, and the pressure is 10 s, respectively, and the chromatogram is recorded. In addition, 1 tablet of recemate amlodipine(labeled with content of 5 mg/ tablet) is taken in a 50 mL volumetric flask, which is soaked for 10 min with ultrasonic aid in appropriate water, and then filters with 0. 45 μm microporous membrane after capacity determination. The content of amlodipine benzenesulfonate is determined by the same method, and the content of

amlodipine benzenesulfonate is calculated according to the peak area by the external standard method.

5 Precautions

(1) Ultrasonic degassing is required before running buffer.

(2) The buffer and sample should be filtered by 0. 45 μm microporous membrane.

(3) When the instrument is operated, the voltage start/stop control button must be pressed. After the high-voltage output is stopped(at this point, the voltage and current are all shown to be 0) , the sampling end of capillary can be taken out.

6 Questions

(1) What are chiral drugs? What are the characteristics of chiral drugs?

(2) What are the characteristics of HPCE?

(3) What are the separation modes of HPCE?

(4) What are the advantages of HPCE, HPLC and GC for the separation of chiral drugs?

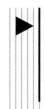

实验十一　咖啡酸片尿药浓度的测定

一、目的要求

（1）了解口服给药的一般方法。
（2）掌握尿样的收集及处理方法。
（3）掌握尿中药物－时间曲线数据的处理方法。

二、实验原理

咖啡酸是一些药用植物中具有止血和升白作用的有效化学成分，其化学名为 3 －（3，4 －二羟基苯基）丙烯酸。其化学合成品已用于临床，一般为其二乙胺盐，以增加其水中溶解度。咖啡酸化学结构如图 2 － 11 － 1 所示。

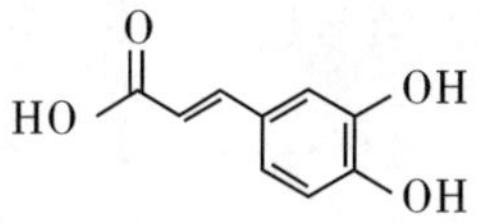

图 2 － 11 － 1　咖啡酸化学结构

本实验根据咖啡酸为酸性药物，从酸化的尿液中用醋酸乙酯提取药物，将提取液蒸发至干，残渣用乙醇溶解，加显色剂显色后，于 520 nm 的波长处进行比色测定。

三、实验仪器与试剂

分光光度计，离心浓缩仪，量筒，10 mL 具塞刻度离心管，10 mL 刻度吸管，显色剂（20% 亚硝酸钠液，20% 铝酸钠溶液，临用前等体积混合），50% 乙醇制氢氧化钠液（2 mol/L），140 μg/mL 咖啡酸对照品水溶液，盐酸，醋酸乙酯，空白尿液。

四、实验步骤

（一）工作曲线的绘制

分别吸取咖啡酸对照品溶液 0 mL、0.2 mL、0.4 mL、0.6 mL、0.8 mL、1.0 mL、1.2 mL，加水（或空白尿）调整体积为 1.2 mL，加盐酸 3 滴，摇匀，加醋酸乙酯

7.0 mL，密塞，振摇 5 min，放置 15 min 使分层（必要时离心）。吸取有机层5.0 mL，置于离心浓缩仪或水浴中，50 ℃减压蒸发至干，放冷，加乙醇（95%）0.5 mL，溶解残渣，再加乙醇制盐酸液（6 mol/L）0.1 mL，显色剂 1.0 mL，充分振摇 1 min，出现黄色混浊，再加50%乙醇制氢氧化钠（2 mol/L）5.0 mL，振摇后混浊消失，溶液显红色，于 520 nm 的波长处测定吸收度。以吸收度为纵坐标、浓度为横坐标绘制工作曲线或计算回归方程。

（二）体内试验

1. 服药方法

健康成年受试者于清晨（空腹）排出第一次晨尿后，饮水100 mL，再排出一次尿，并立即饮水 100 mL，40 min 后接收空白尿（测量总体积），然后用 100 mL 水吞服咖啡酸片 1 片（每片 100 mg），于服药后 0～40 min，40～80 min，80～120 min，120～160 min，160～200 min，200～240 min 接收尿样，并测量各个时间间隔内的尿样总体积，每次接收尿样后都应立即饮水 100 mL，另外，服药 80 min 接收尿样后，进食并补充水分。

2. 尿药浓度的测定

分别吸取空白尿及服药后各时间间隔的尿样各 1.0 mL，加空白尿（或水）0.2 mL，按工作曲线项下，自"加盐酸 3 滴……"起，依法操作，测定的吸收度从工作曲线（或回归方程）读出（或计算）尿药浓度，并乘以尿样体积，即得尿药量，并按"尿药亏量法"计算药物动力学参数。

五、结果处理

已知尿中药物按单房室模型排出的动力学模型为

$$\log \left(X_u^\infty - X_u^t \right) = \log \frac{X_u^\infty K_a}{K_a - K} - \frac{K_t}{2.303}$$

式中，X_u^∞ 为累计排出总药量，X_u^t 为 t 时间累计排出总药量，K_a 为吸收速率常数，K 为消除速率常数。

设在 0～40 min、40～80 min、80～120 min、120～160 min、160～200 min、200～240 min 的时间间隔内排出的尿药量分别为 X_1、X_2、X_3、X_4、X_5、X_6，则 $X_u^\infty = X_1 + \cdots X_6$，$X_u^{40} = X_1$，$X_u^{80} = X_1 + X_2$，$X_u^{120} = X_1 + X_2 + X_3$，依次类推，根据 $\log \left(X_u^\infty - X_u^t \right) \sim t$ 作图，斜率为 $-K/2.303$，并以此可计算 $t_{1/2}$（半衰期）及吸收速率常数。

六、预习提要

（1）尿样处理时应注意哪些问题？

（2）简述"尿药亏量法"计算动力学参数的原理。

（3）显色剂由 20%亚硝酸钠、20%铝酸钠在临用前等量混合制成，为什么？

七、注意事项

（一）实验操作要求

（1）本次实验前，要求学生事先将所用仪器洗净，干燥待用。

（2）实验前一天，受试者服药并收集尿样，服药及收集尿样应按规定程序严格进行。尿样收集后，置冰箱保存。

（3）在测定过程中，醋酸乙酯提取液的蒸发宜在 $50 \sim 60\ ℃$ 的离心浓缩仪或水浴中减压进行，温度过高，有可能造成咖啡酸的氧化分解。加显色剂后若出现浑浊，应离心使溶液澄清，取上清液测定。

（4）若尿药浓度过高，在工作曲线的范围外，应用水或空白尿稀释后测定。

（二）数据处理

尿药数据按单房室模型处理，可用作图法或回归方程计算。有关的原理可参阅药物动力学专著。据文献报道，咖啡酸的 $t_{1/2}$ 约为 $0.67\ h$。

（三）时间安排

本次实验的时间为 5 h 实验课时，宜 2 人一组（视实验条件定），预先安排男同学数名在实验前一天服药、收集尿样。

（四）实验时应注意的问题及解决方法

（1）尿（空白）样贮藏时间不宜过长，否则尿样会出现絮状沉淀。咖啡酸对照品溶液应置冰箱贮藏，以免发霉。

（2）测定过程中，乙酸乙酯蒸干后，试管底部出现不溶于乙醇的沉淀，显色后成颗粒状，影响比色测定，这可能由于试管不洁、显色剂过早混合、尿药浓度过高或温度过高所致，因此应严格控制测定条件。

（3）个别受试者的空白尿样的读数可能高于服药后尿样的读数。

Experiment 11　Determination of Caffeic Acid Concentration in Urine

1　Purposes

(1) To understand the general method of oral administration.

(2) To grasp the urine sample collection and treatment methods.

(3) To grasp the method of processing data in drug-time curve of urine.

2　Principles

Caffeic acid is an effective chemical component with hemostasis and the effect of increasing white blood cell in some medicinal plants. Its synthetics have been used for clinical, which is generally used its diethylamine salt to increase solubility in water. Its chemical name is 3-(3,4-dihydroxyphenyl) acrylic acid(Fig. 2 – 11 – 1) .

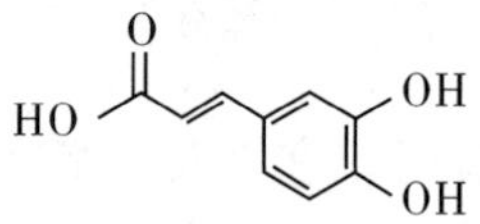

Fig. 2 – 11 – 1　Chemical structure of caffeic acid

According to the fact that caffeic acid is an acidic drug, the drug was extracted from the acidified urine with ethyl acetate. Evaporate the extract to dry, dissolve the residue with ethanol, add chromogenic agent to develop color, then carry out colorimetric determination at the wavelength of 520 nm.

3　Instruments and Reagents

Spectrophotometer, centrifugal concentrator, measuring cylinder, 10 mL centrifuge tube with plug, 10 mL scale pipette.

Chromogenic agent(20% sodium nitrite solution, 20% sodium aluminate solution, mixed in equal volume before use) 50% ethanol sodium hydroxide solution(2 mol/L) , 140 μg/mL caffeic acid reference solution, hydrochloric acid, ethyl acetate, blank urine.

4　Procedures

4.1　Draw Working Curves

Measure 0 mL, 0.2 mL, 0.4 mL, 0.6 mL, 0.8 mL, 1.0 mL, 1.2 mL of standard solutions of caffeic acid, add water(or blank urine) to adjust volume to 1.2 mL, add 3 drops of hydrochloric acid, shake well, add 7.0 mL of ethyl acetate, cover the plug tightly, then shake for 5 min, stand for 15 min to layer(centrifuge if necessary). Take 5.0 mL of organic layer, place it into the test tube on the centrifugal concentrator(or on a water bath) , evaporate the solvent under the negative pressure, cool, add 0.5 mL of ethanol(95%) , dissolve the residue, then add 0. 1 mL of hydrochloric acid(6 mol/L) in ethanol and 1. 0 mL chromogenic agent, shake fully for 1 minute, a yellow turbidity is produced, add 5. 0 mL of sodium hydroxide solution(2 mol/L) in ethanol, the turbidity disappears after shaking and a red color is produced, determine the absorbance of the solution at the wavelength of 520 nm, and draw the working curve or calculate the regression equation with the absorbance as the ordinate against the concentration as the abscissa.

4. 2   Test in Vivo

4. 2. 1   Methods of Taking Medicine

Healthy adult subjects drink 100 mL of water after the first morning urine elimination in the morning(fasting). Urinate again, drink 100 mL of water immediately, after 40 min, collect blank urine(measure total volume), then swallow one caffeic acid tablet(100 mg/ tablet) with 100 mL water. Urine samples are collected for a period of 0 ~ 40 min, 40 ~ 80 min, 80 ~ 120 min, 120 ~ 160 min, 160 ~ 200 min, 200 ~ 240 min after dosing, the total volume at each interval measured. Drink 100 mL of water immediately after each urine sample is collected. In addition, eat and drink water after collecting a urine sample that is collected after taking medicine for 80 min.

4. 2. 2   Determination of Urine Concentration

Take 1. 0 mL of the blank urine and urine samples of each pair of time intervals after taking medicine respectively, add 0. 2 mL of blank urine(or water), operate the experiment since "add three drops of hydrochloric acid…" according to the item of working curve, measure the absorbance, calculate the drug concentration in urine from the working curve (or regression equation), multiply by the volume of the urine sample, and get the amount of drug in urine. Calculate the pharmacokinetic parameters according to "sigma-minus method".

5   Results Processing

The known kinetic model of drug excretion in urine according to the single compartment model is

$$\log \ (X_u^\infty - X_u^t) \ = \log \frac{X_u^\infty K_a}{K_a - K} - \frac{K_t}{2.303}$$

where X_u^∞ is the cumulative total amount of drugs, X_u^t is the cumulative total amount of drugs eliminated at t time, K_a is the absorption rate constant, K is the elimination rate constant.

Suppose the urine drug output is respectively X_1, X_2, X_3, X_4, X_5 and X_6 in the time interval of 0 ~ 40 min, 40 ~ 80 min, 80 ~ 120 min, 120 ~ 160 min, 160 ~ 200 min, 200 ~ 240 min, in that case

$$X_u^\infty = X_1 + \cdots + X_6, X_u^{40} = X_1, \quad X_u^{80} = X_1 + X_2, \quad X_u^{120} = X_1 + X_2 + X_3$$

On the analogy of this, plot according to log $(X_u^\infty - X_u^t) \sim t$, and the slope is $- K/2.303$, $t_{1/2}$ (half-life) and constant absorption rate can be calculated in turn.

6 Previews

(1) What should be paid attention to when treating urine samples?

(2) Briefly describe the computational dynamics parameters of "sigma-minus method".

(3) Chromogenic agent is used after isovolumetric mixing by 20% sodium nitrite solution and 20% sodium aluminate solution before use. Why?

7 Precautions

7.1 Requirements for Experimental Operation

(1) Before this experiment, students are required to wash and dry the instruments to use in advance.

(2) On the day before the experiment, subjects will take medicine and collect urine samples, which should be carried out strictly according to the prescribed procedure. After collecting urine samples, store at the refrigerator.

(3) In the determination process, the evaporation of ethyl acetate extract should be carried out in the water bath at $50 \sim 60$ ℃ with decompression. If the temperature is too high, it may cause the oxidative degradation of caffeic acid. Turbidity occurs after adding chromogenic agent, the solution should be cleared by centrifugation, and the supernatant should be taken for determination.

(4) If the urine concentration is too high, such as outside the scope of the working curve, it should be determined after dilution with water or blank urine.

7.2 Data Processing

The data of urine drug are processed according to the single compartment model, which can be calculated by drawing method or regression equation. The relevant principles are referred to the pharmacokinetics monograph. It has been reported in the literature that the half-life of caffeic acid is about 0.67 h.

7.3 Time Arrangement

The experiment is last for 5 h, it should be 2 students in a group (depending on the experimental conditions), several male students are arranged to take medicine and collect urine samples before the experiment.

7.4 Problems and Solutions in the Experiment

(1) The storage time of urine (blank) sample should not be too long, otherwise there will be flocculent precipitation in urine sample. Caffeic acid reference solution should also be stored in the refrigerator, in order to avoid mildew phenomenon.

(2) During the determination process, after ethyl acetate is dried, the insoluble ethanol precipitate appeared at the bottom of the test tube, graininess appears after color development, which affects the colorimetric determination, it may be due to unclean test

tube, premature mixing of chromogenic agents, excessive urine concentration and excessive temperature, so the determination conditions should be strictly controlled.

(3) The reading of blank urine sample is higher than the reading of urine sample after taking medicine for individual subjects.

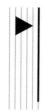

实验十二　兔血浆中茶碱血药浓度的高效液相色谱法分析

一、目的要求

（1）掌握高效液相色谱法测定茶碱血药浓度的方法。

（2）掌握家兔静脉给药的方法。

（3）掌握血样的收集及前处理方法。

（4）掌握房室模型的判断及相关药代动力学参数的计算方法。

二、实验原理

茶碱化学结构如图 2 - 12 - 1 所示，茶碱是甲基嘌呤类药物，具有扩张冠状动脉、强心、利尿、松弛支气管平滑肌和兴奋中枢神经系统等作用，是临床上常用的支气管扩张药，可直接松弛气道平滑肌，用于慢性哮喘的维持治疗及其他慢性阻塞性肺病等引发的可逆性气道阻塞的治疗。茶碱的治疗血药浓度较窄（5 ～ 20 μg/mL）。茶碱血浆浓度 <5 μg/mL 时几乎无药效反应，5 ～ 10 μg/mL 有效，10 ～ 20 μg/mL 达最佳疗效，>20 μg/mL 即有毒性反应表现，30 ～ 40 μg/mL 时可引起严重中毒反应，且个体差异很大，血中的浓度较难控制，故易发生中毒。凡接受茶碱类药物治疗的患者在有条件时均应进行血药浓度监测。

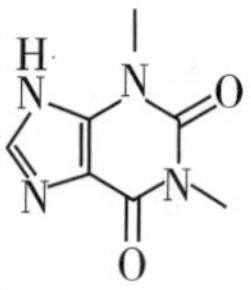

图 2 - 12 - 1　茶碱的化学结构

本品为白色结晶性粉末，在乙醇和三氯甲烷中微溶，在水中极微溶解，在乙醚中几乎不溶；在氢氧化钠溶液或氨溶液中易溶。茶碱具有较强的紫外吸收，在 271 nm 有最大吸收。血浆中的茶碱在微酸性溶液中，可用乙酸乙酯提取，分取乙酸乙酯提取液，水浴氮气吹干或真空干燥箱 50 ℃以下脱去溶剂，残渣加流动相溶解，离心，取上清液进样。由于本品提取步骤较多，易引入误差，为此采用内标法。

生物样品中通常除含有药物外，还含有该药物的一种或多种代谢产物及体内的内源性物质，测定样品中药物含量时，杂质会干扰测定，因此必须对被测物质进行提取、分离、纯化、浓集或衍生化处理。生物样品经预处理后，得到较纯的含药物的萃取物，便于后续分析。内标法主要用于校正生物样品从萃取到色谱分离过程中各种因素导致的药物损失，提高分析结果的精密度和准确度。

用作内标的化合物或药物的物理化学性质必须与待测物质的物理化学性质非常相似，且内标和待测成分具有相同的热稳定性，内标的选择原则见实验七。

三、实验仪器与试剂

（一）仪器
高效液相色谱仪，漩涡混合器，离心机，注射器（10 mL），家兔固定木盒，红外灯，灌胃器，刀片，2 mL 离心管，5 mL 离心管等。

（二）试剂
家兔（体重约 2.5 kg，实验前禁食一夜），茶碱对照品，茶碱水溶液（15 mg/mL），1，3 - 二硝基苯（内标），肝素，乙酸乙酯。

四、实验步骤

（一）溶液的配制
茶碱对照品溶液：取茶碱对照品约 100 mg，精密称定，置 100 mL 量瓶中，用水溶解，稀释成 1 000 μg/mL 的对照品储备液，精密量取茶碱对照品储备液适量，用水稀释成浓度分别为 2.00 μg/mL、5.00 μg/mL、10.00 μg/mL、20.00 μg/mL、30.00 μg/mL、50.00 μg/mL、100.00 μg/mL 的茶碱系列对照品溶液，4 ℃冷藏备用。

1，3 - 二硝基苯内标溶液：取 1，3 - 二硝基苯约 10 mg，精密称定，置 100 mL 量瓶中，用乙酸乙酯溶解，并定量稀释成含 1，3 - 二硝基苯 100 μg/mL 的溶液，精密量取该溶液 1 mL 至 100 mL 量瓶中，用乙酸乙酯稀释至 1 μg/mL 的内标溶液，4 ℃冷藏。

（二）给药方法及样品采集
取体重约为 2.5 kg 的健康家兔，在非给药侧耳朵耳缘静脉处把毛剪去，使静脉显露。每次取血前用灯照几分钟，灯照下耳血管充分充盈后，在耳缘静脉处将皮切开一个小口，露出静脉，把静脉切开一半（不要切断），血液从切口处流出，置于含有肝素的 2 mL 离心管中（取血前用棉签蘸取肝素粉末适量，直接涂撒在离心管内壁），加入血样后立即轻轻旋摇，勿太猛烈，以免导致红细胞破裂。离心分取上层淡黄色液体，即得空白血浆。取血毕，用棉花置于切口，轻压，防止出血。下次取血前用干棉球轻揉切口，抹去血痂，即可取血，不必另做切口。

从兔耳静脉快速注射茶碱水溶液（15 mg/mL）1 mL，分别于给药后 5 min、15 min、30 min 及 1 h、2 h、3 h、4 h、6 h、8 h 从耳静脉取血约 0.4 mL，分取血浆置冰箱保存备用。

（三）茶碱血浆样品处理

取冷冻的血浆样品，室温解冻，精密吸取 100 μL，置 5 mL 离心管中，加水 100 μL，混匀，在 37 ℃ 水浴中保温 30 min，精密加入 1，3 - 二硝基苯内标溶液 1 mL，涡旋混合 3 min，3 000 转/分离心 10 min，分取上层有机相 0.8 mL，置于另一 2 mL 离心管中，50 ℃ 真空干燥箱中减压挥干溶剂，残渣加 100 μL 流动相涡旋，溶解，离心，取上清液 10 μL 进样。

（四）茶碱血浆标准曲线

取空白血浆 100 μL，分别置于 5 mL 离心管中，精密加入每毫升含茶碱 2.00 μg/mL、5.00 μg/mL、10.00 μg/mL、20.00 μg/mL、30.00 μg/mL、50.00 μg/mL、100.00 μg/mL 的对照品溶液各 100 μL，涡旋混合 5 s，在 37 ℃ 水浴中保温 30 min，按 "（三）茶碱血浆样品处理"，自 "精密加入 1，3 - 二硝基苯内标溶液 1 mL" 起，同法处理，进样 10 μL，记录色谱图。以茶碱血浆浓度为横坐标，茶碱与内标的峰面积比值为纵坐标，用加权（$W = 1/x^2$）最小二乘法进行线性回归，求得的直线方程即为标准曲线。

（五）血浆中茶碱血药浓度的 HPLC 测定

照高效液相色谱法［《中国药典》（2020 年版）通则 0512］测定。

色谱条件：色谱柱：ODS C18 色谱柱（4.6 mm×250 mm，10 μm）；流动相：甲醇—水（50：50）；流速：1.0 mL/min；检测波长：254 nm。取空白血浆样品和 "（四）茶碱血浆标准曲线" 项下血浆对照品样品（30.0 μg/mL）分别测定，茶碱与 1，3 - 二硝基苯（内标）的分离度应大于 1.5，空白血浆样品色谱图中，在茶碱与内标位置应没有干扰峰。

测定法：取含药血浆样品供试液 10 μL，注入液相色谱仪，记录色谱图，按内标法用标准曲线计算即得。

（六）药动学参数计算

房室模型的判断：对一个药物的药代动力学参数进行分析计算时，首先要确定该药在体内的运转是符合一室模型还是二室模型。常用的图解法是一个实用的判断方法。将血药浓度的实验数据对时间在半对数纸上作图（浓度为纵坐标）。如果各实验点可连成一条直线，属于一室模型，按一级动力学从血中清除。如果药时曲线可连成两段直线，属于二室模型。这时，根据图解和开放性二室模型的公式，计算各项药代动力学参数，二室药时曲线呈双指数衰减。前一段直线主要反应分布过程，称分布相或 α 相；后一段直线主要反映分布平衡后进入缓慢消除过程，称消除相或 β 相。

参数计算：房室模型确定后计算相应的药代动力学参数。

五、预习提要

（1）家兔取血时应注意哪些问题？

（2）血浆与血清有什么区别？如何制备血浆样品？

（3）血样采集及血样处理应注意哪些问题？

（4）常用的血浆样品前处理方法有哪些？

（5）一般药物含量测定常采用最小二乘法进行线性回归，为什么血浆样品标准曲线要采用加权最小二乘法进行线性回归？

（6）一室模型与二室模型有何区别？一室模型或二室模型的相应参数计算请参照《生物药剂学与药物动力学》课本第二编第二章、第三章相关内容。

六、注意事项

（1）本次实验前，要熟悉高效液相色谱仪的使用。

（2）若血药浓度过高，在工作曲线的范围外，应用空白血浆稀释后测定。

（3）取血时要注意不要发生溶血。

（4）萃取溶剂挥干并用流动相复溶时，常会出现浑浊现象（脂肪类物质未完全溶解），此时应该离心后取上清液进样，保护色谱柱。

（5）在非给药侧耳朵耳缘静脉取血样，切勿在同侧取血。

Experiment 12　Determination of Theophylline in Rabbit's Plasma by HPLC

1　Purposes

(1) To master the method of determining theophylline plasma concentration by HPLC.

(2) To master the method of intravenous injection in rabbits.

(3) To master the methods for collection and pretreatment of blood samples.

(4) To master the judgment of atrioventricular model and the calculation method of related pharmacokinetic parameters.

2　Principles

The chemical structure of theophylline is shown in Fig. 2 – 12 – 1. It is a methylpurine drug. It has the functions of dilating coronary artery, strengthening heart, diuresis, relaxing bronchial smooth muscle and exciting central nervous system. It is a commonly used bronchodilator in clinic. It can directly relax the musle of respiratory tract and is used for maintenance treatment of chronic asthma and reversible respiratory tract obstruction caused by other chronic obstructive pulmonary diseases. Theophylline has a narrow plasma concentration(5 ~ 20 μg/mL). When the concentration of theophylline in plasma is less than 5 μg/mL, there is almost no pharmacodynamic response; 5 ~ 10 μg/mL is effective; 10 ~ 20 μg/mL is the best. When the concentration of theophylline is more than 20 μg/mL, there is toxic reaction. When the concentration of theophylline reaches 30 ~ 40 μg/mL, it could cause serious toxic reaction, and the individual difference is very big, the blood concentration is difficult to be controlled, so it is prone to poisoning. The concentration of theophylline in plasma should be monitored for those patients receiving theophylline therapy, when conditions permit.

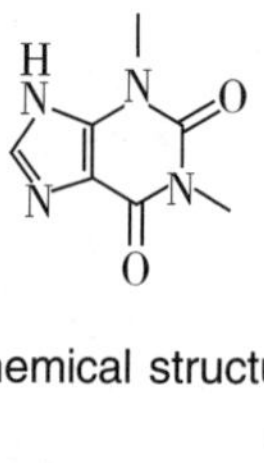

Fig. 2 – 12 – 1　Chemical structure of theophylline

Theophylline is a white crystalline powder, slightly soluble in ethanol and chloroform, very slightly soluble in water, almost insoluble in ether; easily soluble in sodium hydroxide solution or ammonia solution. Theophylline has a strong UV absorption and the maximum absorption at 271 nm. Theophylline in plasma can be extracted with ethyl acetate. The ethyl acetate extract is separated and dried in water bath with nitrogen or under vacuum condition in vacuum drying oven below 50 ℃. The residue is dissolved with mobile phase, centrifuged and the supernatant is injected. Because there are many steps to extract this product, it is easy to introduce errors, so the internal standard method is used.

In addition to drugs, biological samples usually contain one or more metabolites of the drug and endogenous substances in the body. Impurities will interfere the determination of the drug content in the samples, so it is necessary to extract, separate, purify, concentrate or derive the tested substances. After pretreatment of biological samples, a pure extract containing drugs is obtained, which is convenient for subsequent analysis. Internal standard method is mainly used to correct the drug loss caused by various factors in the process of biological samples from extraction to chromatographic separation, and improve the precision and accuracy of analytical results.

The physical and chemical properties of the compounds or drugs to be used as internal standards must be very similar to those of the substances to be tested, and the internal standards and the components to be tested have the same thermal stability. The general selection principles on how to choose an internal standard can be consulted in Experiment 7.

3 Instruments and Reagents

3.1 Instruments

High performance liquid chromatograph, whirlpool mixer, centrifuge, syringe(10 mL), rabbit fixed wooden box, infrared lamp, gastric irrigator, blade, 2 mL centrifuge tube, 5 mL centrifuge tube, etc.

3.2 Reagents

Rabbits(weight about 2.5 kg, fasting one night before the experiment), theophylline reference substance, theophylline aqueous solution(15 mg/mL), 1,3-dinitrobenzene(internal standard), heparin.

4 Procedures

4.1 Preparation of Solution

Theophylline Reference Solution: Take about 100 mg of theophylline reference solution, accurately weighed, put it into a 100 mL volumetric flask, dissolve with water, dilute it containing 1 000 μg/mL as theophylline reference stock solution, accurately measure an appropriate amount of theophylline reference stock solution, dilute it with water into a series of reference solutions with concentration of 2.00 μg/mL, 5.00 μg/mL, 10.00 μg/mL, 20.00 μg/mL, 30.00 μg/mL, 50.00 μg/mL and 100.00 μg/mL respectively, and store them under 4 ℃ for future use.

1,3-Dinitrobenzene Internal Standard Solution: Take about 10mg of 1,3-dinitrobenzene, accurately weighed, put it into a 100 mL volumetric flask, dissolve it with ethyl acetate, and quantitatively dilute it into a solution containing 100 μg/mL of 1,3-dinitrobenzene. Precisely measure the solution in a 1 mL to 100 mL volumetric flask, dilute it with ethyl acetate to 1 μg/mL of internal standard solution, and refrigerate at 4 ℃.

4.2　Administration Method and Sample Collection

A healthy rabbit weighing about 2.5 kg is selected. The hair is cut off at the vein of the ear margin of the non drug side to expose the vein. Each time before taking blood, light it for a few minutes with a lamp. After the ear blood vessels are fully filled with the heat of the lamp, cut a small incision in the vein of the ear edge to expose the vein. Cut half of the vein (do not cut it off). The blood flows out from the incision and is placed in a 2 mL centrifuge tube containing heparin(before taking blood, use a cotton swab to dip an appropriate amount of heparin powder and directly spread it on the inner wall of the centrifuge tube). After sampling, gently rotate and shake immediately, not too violently, so as not to cause the red blood cells to break. The upper layer of pale yellow liquid is centrifuged to obtain blank plasma. After taking the blood, put the cotton on the incision and press it gently to prevent bleeding. Before the next blood collection, gently rub the incision with a dry cotton ball and wipe off the blood scab to get blood without making another incision.

1 mL of theophylline solution(15 mg/mL) is injected into the ear vein of rabbits rapidly. About 0.4 mL blood is taken from the ear vein at 5 min, 15 min, 30 min and 1 h, 2 h, 3 h, 4 h, 6 h, 8 h after administration, respectively. The plasma is separated and stores in the refrigerator.

4.3　Treatment of Theophylline Plasma Samples

Take the frozen plasma samples, thaw it at room temperature, accurately take 100 μL, put it in a 5 mL centrifuge tube, add 100 μL water, mix well, keep it on a 37 ℃ water bath for 30 min, and add 1 mL of 1,3-dinitrobenzene internal standard solution, vortex mixing for 3 min, centrifugate at 3 000 rpm for 10 min, separate 0.8 mL of upper organic phase, put it in another 2 mL centrifuge tube, evaporate the solvent under reduced pressure below 50 ℃ in vacuum drying oven, add 100 μL mobile phase vortex the residue, dissolve, centrifuge, and take 10 μL supernatant for injection.

4.4　Theophylline Standard Curve in Plasma

Measure 100 μL blank plasma and put it in a 5 mL centrifuge tube, precisely add 100 μL control solution containing 2.00 μL/mL, 5.00 μL/mL, 10.00 μL/mL, 20.00 μL/mL, 30.00 μL/mL, 50.00 μL/mL and 100.00 μL/mL theophylline, respectively, mix it on vortex for 5 s, keep it in water bath at 37 ℃ for 30 min, do it according to "Treatment of Theophylline Plasma Samples", then add it from "and add 1 mL of 1,3-dinitrobenzene internal standard solution", treat it with the same method, inject 10 μL, and record the chromatogram. Take theophylline plasma concentration as abscissa and the ratio of peak area of theophylline to internal standard as ordinate, the linear regression is carried out by weighted($W = 1/x^2$) least square method, and the linear equation obtained as the standard curve.

4. 5　Determination of Theophylline in Plasma by HPLC

Carry out the method for HPLC (General Rule 0512), using a column (4. 6 mm × 250 mm, 10 μm) packed with octadecyl silane and a mixture of methanol-water (50 : 50) as the mobile phase; the flow rate is 1. 0 mL/min; and the detection wavelength is set at 254 nm. The blank plasma sample and the calibration curve solution which contains 30. 0 μg/mL theophylline are determined separately, and the peak responses are recorded. The resolution between theophylline and 1, 3-dinitrobenzene(internal standard) should be greater than 1. 5. In the chromatogram of blank plasma sample, there should be no interference peak at the retention time of theophylline and internal standard.

Determinaion: A portion of the supernatant(10 μL) is injected into HPLC system and the chromatogram is recorded. The concentration of theophylline in plasma is calculated according to standard curve by internal standard method.

4. 6　Calculation of Pharmacokinetic Parameters

When analyzing and calculating the pharmacokinetic parameters of a drug, it is necessary to accurately determine whether the drug is in accordance with the one compartment model or the two compartment model. The commonly used graphic method is a practical judgment method. The experimental data of blood concentration are plotted on semi logarithmic paper(the concentration is ordinate). If each experimental point can be connected into a straight line, it belongs to a one compartment model and is removed from the blood according to the first-order kinetics. If the drug time curve can be connected into two straight lines, it belongs to two compartment model. At this time, according to the diagram and the formula of the open two compartment model, the kinetic parameters are calculated, and the two compartment drug time curve shows double exponential decay. The first straight line mainly reflects the distribution process, which is called distribution phase or α phase; the second straight line mainly reflects the distribution equilibrium and then enters the slow elimination process, which is called elimination phase or β phase.

The pharmacokinetic parameters are calculated after the atrioventricular model is determined.

5　Previews

(1) What problems should be paid attention to when taking blood from rabbits?

(2) What is the difference between plasma and serum? How to prepare plasma samples?

(3) What problems should be paid attention to in blood sample collection and blood sample processing?

(4) What are the common used pretreatment methods for plasma samples?

(5) In general, the least square method is often used for linear regression in the determination of drug content. Why should the weighted least square method be used for linear regression in the standard curve of plasma samples?

(6) What is the difference between one compartment model and two compartment model? Please refer to Chapter 2 and Chapter 3 of *Biopharmaceutics and Pharmacokinetics* for the calculation of corresponding parameters of one compartment model or two compartment model.

6 Precautions

(1) Be familiar with the use of HPLC before this experiment.

(2) If the plasma concentration is too high, and is outside the range of the standard curve, the blank plasma should be used for dilution and determination.

(3) Take all feasible measures and methods to avoid hemolysis when blood is taken.

(4) When redissolve the residue after the extraction solvent is volatilized with mobile phase, the turbid phenomenon often occurs (the fatty substances are not completely dissolved) . At this time, the supernatant should be taken for injection after centrifugation to protect the chromatographic column.

(5) Blood samples shound be taken from the ear marginal vein of the ear on the non-administration side. Do not take blood on the same ear.

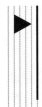

实验十三　设计性实验——对乙酰氨基酚片的含量测定

一、目的要求

（1）掌握对乙酰氨基酚片含量测定的基本原理。

（2）学会根据实验目的要求查阅相关文献。

（3）根据对乙酰氨基酚的化学结构及查阅的文献，选择适当的实验方法，对其进行含量测定。

（4）根据《中国药典》（2020 年版）通则 9101 分析方法验证指导原则，对设计的对乙酰氨基酚片含量测定方法进行验证。

（5）能够根据实验设计进行操作，得出实验结论。

（6）掌握含量测定方法验证的内容。

（7）掌握常用药物含量测定方法的基本操作及药物含量的计算方法。

（8）培养独立分析问题、解决问题的能力及实际动手能力。

二、实验试剂

对乙酰氨基酚片等。

三、实验步骤

（1）根据对乙酰氨基酚的化学结构、理化特性，以及查阅的相关文献，选择适当方法，设计合理的实验流程，对其进行含量测定。

（2）实验前应写出实验设计报告，其内容及格式可参考"实验三：苯甲酸钠的分析"相关内容。设计报告必须包括以下内容：仪器及试药、实验准备、实验方法、注意事项、参考文献。其他有必要或有意义的内容可酌情添加。

（3）根据实验的内容和目的，参照实验"实验三　苯甲酸钠的分析"的相关内容，设计原始记录和检验报告。

（4）按照实验设计准备实验，开展实验，测定对乙酰氨基酚片的含量，做好原始记录，计算对乙酰氨基酚片的含量，得出实验结论，写出实验报告。

（5）实验结束后，根据本次实验情况写一份实验总结，包括含量测定方法学验证。

四、注意事项

（1）设计实验前应充分了解对乙酰氨基酚的理化特性，选择最恰当的方法测定其含量。文献查阅时，对该药物的各种相关分析方法应进行检索，如不同剂型的分析方法、各种生物样本中的分析方法等。

（2）设计实验时应尽量选择最佳方法，以求简便、快速、低耗地得出正确可靠的实验结果。

（3）实验设计报告中的仪器及试剂主要指实验中所要应用的器材、试剂、药品、对照品、标准品等。实验准备主要指实验中所要应用的滴定液、缓冲液、溶液、试液、试纸、指示液等的配制。实验方法主要指实验的操作步骤及方法，应写清其实验原理，总的来说应写得明了、清楚，同时尽量简洁。注意事项主要指实验中应格外注意，操作不当易导致实验误差，严重时甚至会引起实验事故的一些问题。参考文献指实验设计中主要参考的文献著作，应注意其书写格式。

（4）原始记录及检验报告均应设计合理。原始记录：各重要原始数据、实验现象均应有相应的足够的地方记录，切不可疏漏，也应避免繁复；实验报告：相应数据、计算、结果、结论及必要的图表等均应记录，同样应避免疏漏、繁复。

（5）实验总结的书写内容：评价实验设计报告、原始记录及检验报告有何优点及不妥之处，在实验中发现了哪些问题，可以怎样改善，以及其他认为值得讨论的问题。

五、思考题

除了最终选择的实验方法外，还有哪些方法可以选择？为何在各种方法中选择该法测定药物含量？其优越性何在？

Experiment 13　Design Experiment—Determination of Acetaminophen Tablets

1　Purposes

（1）To master the basic principle of determination of acetaminophen tablets.

（2）To consult relevant literature according to the requirements of experiment purposes.

（3）To select appropriate experimental methods to determine the content according to the chemical structure of acetaminophen and the literature.

（4）To valid the method adopted for the determination of acetaminophen tablets according to the General Rule：9101 for Validation of Analytical Method, recorded in *Chinese Pharmacopoeia* （2020 edition）.

（5）To operate the experiment according to the experimental design and draw a conclusion.

（6）To master the content for validation of analytical method in determination of content.

（7）To master the basic operation of common drug determination methods and calculation methods of drug content.

（8）To develop the ability of independent analysis, problem solving and practical ability.

2　Reagents

Acetaminophen tablets, etc.

3　Procedures

（1）According to the chemical structure, physical and chemical characteristics of acetaminophen and relevant literature, select appropriate methods, design reasonable experimental procedures and determine its content.

（2）The experiment design report should be written before the experiment. The content and format can be referred to the related content of Experiment 3. The design report should include the following contents：instruments and test drugs, experimental preparation, experimental methods, precautions, and references. Other necessary and meaningful content may be added as appropriate.

（3）According to the content and purposes of the experiment, refer to the related content of Experiment 3, and design the original record and inspection report.

（4）Prepare the experiment according to the experiment design, carry out the experiment, determine the content of acetaminophen tablets, make the original record, calculate the content of acetaminophen tablets, draw the test conclusion, and write the test

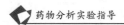

report.

(5) After the experiment, write a summary of the experiment according to the situation of the experiment, including methodology verification.

4 Precautions

(1) Before designing the experiment, fully understand the physical and chemical characteristics of acetaminophen, and choose the most appropriate method to determine its content. In the literature review, various related analysis methods of the drug should be searched, such as analysis methods of different dosage forms and analysis methods in various biological samples.

(2) The optimal method should be selected as far as possible in the design of experiments, to obtain correct and reliable experimental results in a simple, rapid and low-cost manner.

(3) The instruments and reagents in the experimental design report mainly refer to the equipment, reagents, drugs, reference and standard products to be used in the experiment. Experimental preparation mainly refers to the preparation of titrate, buffer, solution, test solution, test paper, indicator, etc. The experimental method mainly refers to the operation steps and methods of the experiment, and its experimental principle should be clearly written. Precautions mainly refer to the extra attention to be paid to in the experiment. Improper operation can easily lead to experimental error, and even cause some problems of experimental accident in serious cases. Reference refers to the main reference works in experimental design, and should pay attention to its writing format.

(4) Original records and inspection reports shall be properly designed. Original records: All important raw data and experimental phenomena should be recorded in adequate places, avoid omission and complexity. Inspection report: the corresponding data, calculation, results, conclusions and necessary charts should be recorded, and should avoid omission and complexity.

(5) Contents of the experiment summary: Evaluate the advantages and disadvantages of the experiment design report, original record and inspection report, find out the problems in the experiment and how to improve them, and other issues worth discussing.

5 Questions

In addition to the final experimental method, what other methods can be selected? Why choose the method for the determination of drug content in various methods? What advantages are there?

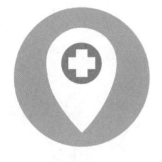

附　　录

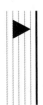

附录一　《中国药典》（2020 年版）
通则 9101　分析方法验证指导原则

　　分析方法验证（analytical method validation）的目的是证明建立的方法适合于相应检测要求。在建立药品质量标准、变更药品生产工艺或制剂组分、修订原分析方法时，需要对分析方法进行验证。生物制品质量控制中采用的方法包括理化分析方法和生物学测定方法，其中理化分析方法的验证原则与化学药品基本相同，所以可参照本指导原则进行，但在进行具体验证时还需要结合生物制品的特点考虑；相对于理化分析方法而言，生物学测定方法存在更多的影响因素，因此，本指导原则不涉及生物学测定方法验证的内容。

　　验证的分析项目有：鉴别试验、杂质测定（限度或定量分析）、含量测定（包括特性参数和含量/效价测定，其中特性参数如：药物溶出度、释放度等）。

　　验证的指标有：专属性、准确度、精密度（包括重复性、中间精密度和重现性）、检测限、定量限、线性、范围和耐用性。在分析方法验证中，须用标准物质进行试验。由于分析方法具有各自的特点，并随分析对象而变化，因此需要视具体情况拟订验证的指标。表 1 中列出的分析项目和相应的验证指标可供参考。

表 1　检验项目和验证指标

参数	鉴别	杂质测定		含量测定—特性参数—含量或效价测定
		定量	限度	
准确度	−	+	−	+
精密度				
重复性	−	+	−	+
中间精密度	−	+[①]	−	+[①]
专属性[②]	+	+	+	+
检测限	−	−[③]	+	−
定量限	−	+	−	−
线性	−	+	−	+
范围	−	+	−	+
耐用性	+	+	+	+

　　①已有重现性验证，不需要验证中间精密度。
　　②如一种方法不够专属，可用其他分析方法予以补充。
　　③视具体情况予以验证。

　　方法验证内容如下。

一、专属性

专属性系指在其他成分（如杂质、降解产物、辅料等）可能存在的情况下，采用的分析方法能正确测定出被测物的能力。鉴别反应、杂质检查和含量测定方法，均应考察其专属性。如方法专属性不强，应采用多种不同原理的方法予以补充。

1. 鉴别反应

应能区分可能共存的物质或结构相似的化合物。不含被测成分的供试品，以及结构相似或组分中的有关化合物，应均呈阴性反应。

2. 含量测定和杂质测定

采用的色谱法和其他分离方法，应附代表性图谱，以说明方法的专属性，并应标明各成分在图中的位置，色谱法中的分离度应符合要求。

在杂质对照品可获得的情况下，对于含量测定，试样中可加入杂质或辅料，考察测定结果是否受干扰，并可与未加杂质或辅料的试样比较测定结果。对于杂质检查，也可向试样中加入一定量的杂质，考察各成分包括杂质之间能否得到分离。

在杂质不能获得的情况下，可将含有杂质或降解产物的试样进行测定，与另一个经验证了的方法或药典方法比较结果。也可用强光照射、高温、高湿、酸（碱）水解或氧化的方法进行加速破坏，以研究可能的降解产物和降解途径对含量测定和杂质测定的影响。含量测定方法应比对两种方法的结果，杂质检查应比对检出的杂质个数，必要时可采用光电二极管阵列检测和质谱检测，进行峰纯度检查。

二、准确度

准确度系指用所建立方法测定的结果与真实值或参比值接近的程度，一般用回收率（%）表示。准确度应在规定的线性范围内试验。准确度也可由所测定的精密度、线性和专属性推算出来。

在规定范围内，取同一浓度（相当于100%浓度水平）的供试品，用至少6份样品的测定结果进行评价；或设计至少3种不同浓度，每种浓度分别制备至少3份供试品溶液进行测定，用至少9份样品的测定结果进行评价，且浓度的设定应考虑样品的浓度范围。两种方法的选定应考虑分析的目的和样品的浓度范围。

1. 化学药含量测定方法的准确度

原料药可用已知纯度的对照品或供试品进行测定，或用所测定结果与已知准确度的另一个方法的测定结果进行比较。制剂可在处方量空白辅料中，加入已知量被测物对照品进行测定。如不能得到制剂辅料的全部组分，可向待测制剂中加入已知量的被测物进行测定，或用所建立方法的测定结果与已知准确度的另一个方法的测定结果进行比较。

2. 化学药杂质定量测定的准确度

化学药杂质定量测定的准确度可通过向原料药或制剂处方量空白辅料中加入已知量杂质对照品进行测定。如不能得到杂质对照品，可用所建立的方法测定的结果与另一成熟的方法（如药典标准方法或经过验证的方法）进行比较。

3. 中药化学成分测定方法的准确度

中药化学成分测定方法的准确度可用已知纯度的对照品进行加样回收率测定，即向已知被测成分含量的供试品中再精密加入一定量的已知纯度的被测成分对照品，依法测定。用实测值与供试品中含有量之差，除以加入对照品量计算回收率。在加样回收试验中须注意对照品的加入量与供试品中被测成分含有量之和必须在标准曲线线性范围之内；加入的对照品的量要适当，过小则引起较大的相对误差，过大则干扰成分相对减少，真实性差。

4. 数据要求

对于化学药，应报告已知加入量的回收率（%），或测定结果平均值与真实值之差及其相对标准偏差或置信区间（置信度一般为 95%）；对于中药，应报告供试品取样量、供试品中含有量、对照品加入量、测定结果和回收率（%）计算值，以及回收率（%）的相对标准偏差（RSD,%）或置信区间。样品中待测定成分含量和回收率限度关系可参考表 2。在基质复杂、组分含量低于 0.01% 及多成分等分析中，回收率限度可适当放宽。

表 2　样品中待测定成分含量和回收率限度 *

待测定成分含量			待测定成分质量分数	回收率限度/%
%	ppm 或 ppb	g/mg 或 μg/g	g/g	
100	—	1 000 mg/g	1.0	98～101
10	100 000 ppm	100 mg/g	0.1	95～102
1	10 000 ppm	10 mg/g	0.01	92～105
0.1	1 000 ppm	1 mg/g	0.001	90～108
0.01	100 ppm	100 μg/g	0.000 1	85～110
0.001	10 ppm	10 μg/g	0.000 01	80～115
0.0001	1 ppm	1 μg/g	0.000 001	75～120
—	10 ppb	0.01 μg/g	0.000 000 01	70～125

* 此表源自 AOAC *Guidelines for Single Laboratory Validation of Chemical Methods for Dietary Supplements and Botanicals*。

三、精密度

精密度系指在规定的测定条件下，同一份均匀供试品，经多次取样测定所得结果之间的接近程度。精密度一般用偏差、标准偏差或相对标准偏差表示。在相同条件下，由同一个分析人员测定所得结果的精密度称为重复性；在同一个实验室，不同时间由不同分析人员用不同设备测定结果之间的精密度，称为中间精密度；在不同实验室由不同分析人员测定结果之间的精密度，称为重现性。含量测定和杂质的定量测定应考察方法的精密度。

1. **重复性**

在规定范围内，取同一浓度（分析方法拟定的样品测定浓度，相当于100%浓度水平）的供试品，用至少6份测定结果进行评价；或设计3种不同浓度，每种浓度分别制备3份供试品溶液进行测定，用9份样品的测定结果进行评价。采用9份测定结果进行评价时，浓度的设定应考虑样品的浓度范围。

2. **中间精密度**

考察随机变动因素如不同日期、不同分析人员、不同仪器对精密度的影响，应设计方案进行中间精密度试验。

3. **重现性**

使用国家药品质量标准采用的分析方法，应进行重现性试验，如通过不同实验室协同检验获得重现性结果。协同检验的目的、过程和重现性结果均应记载在起草说明中。应注意重现性试验所用样品质量的一致性及贮存运输中的环境对该一致性的影响，以免影响重现性试验结果。

4. **数据要求**

均应报告偏差、标准偏差、相对标准偏差或置信区间。样品中待测定成分含量和精密度 RSD 可接受范围参考表 3（计算公式，重复性：$RSD_r = C^{-0.15}$；重现性：$RSD_R = 2C^{-0.15}$，其中 C 为待测定成分含量）。在基质复杂、组分含量低于 0.01% 及多成分等分析中，精密度限度可适当放宽。

表 3　样品中待测定成分的含量与精密度可接受范围关系[*]

待测定成分含量			待测定成分质量分数	重复性（RSD）/%	重现性（RSD）/%
%	ppm 或 ppb	g/mg 或 μg/g	g/g		
100	—	1 000 mg/g	1.0	1	2
10	100 000 ppm	100 mg/g	0.1	1.5	3
1	10 000 ppm	10 mg/g	0.01	2	4
0.1	1 000 ppm	1 mg/g	0.001	3	6

续表 3

待测定成分含量			待测定成分质量分数	重复性（RSD）/%	重现性（RSD）/%
%	ppm 或 ppb	g/mg 或 μg/g	g/g		
0.01	100 ppm	100 μg/g	0.000 1	4	8
0.001	10 ppm	10 μg/g	0.000 01	6	11
0.000 1	1 ppm	1 μg/g	0.000 001	8	16
—	10 ppb	0.01 μg/g	0.000 000 01	15	32

＊此表源自 AOAC *Guidelines for Single Laboratory Validation of Chemical Methods for Dietary Supplements and Botanicals*。

四、检测限

检测限系指试样中被测物能被检测出的最低量。检测限仅作为限度试验指标和定性鉴别的依据，没有定量意义。常用的方法如下。

1. 直观法

用已知浓度的被测物，试验出能被可靠地检测出的最低浓度或量。

2. 信噪比法

用于能显示基线噪声的分析方法，即把已知低浓度试样测出的信号与空白样品测出的信号进行比较，计算出能被可靠地检测出的被测物质的最低浓度或量。一般以信噪比为 3∶1 时相应浓度或注入仪器的量确定检测限。

3. 基于响应值标准偏差和标准曲线斜率法

按照 $LOD = 3.3 \, \delta/S$ 公式计算，式中，LOD 为检测限；δ 为响应值的偏差；S 为标准曲线的斜率。δ 可以通过下列方法测得：①测定空白值的标准偏差；②标准曲线的剩余标准偏差或是截距的标准偏差。

4. 数据要求

上述计算方法获得的检测限数据须用含量相近的样品进行验证。应附测定图谱，说明试验过程和检测限结果。

五、定量限

定量限系指试样中被测物能被定量测定的最低量，其测定结果应符合准确度和精密度要求。对微量或痕量药物分析、定量测定药物杂质和降解产物时，应确定方法的定量限。常用的方法如下。

1. 直观法

直观法是用已知浓度的被测物，试验出能被可靠地定量测定的最低浓度或量。

2. 信噪比法

信噪比法是用于能显示基线噪声的分析方法，即将已知低浓度试样测出的信号与空白样品测出的信号进行比较，计算出能被可靠地定量的被测物质的最低浓度或量。一般以信噪比为 10∶1 时的相应浓度或注入仪器的量确定定量限。

3. 基于响应值标准偏差和标准曲线斜率法

按照 $LOQ = 10\,\delta/S$ 公式计算，式中，LOQ 为定量限，δ 为响应值的偏差，S 为标准曲线的斜率。δ 可以通过下列方法测得：①测定空白值的标准偏差；②采用标准曲线的剩余标准偏差或是截距的标准偏差。

4. 数据要求

上述计算方法获得的定量限数据须用含量相近的样品进行验证。应附测试图谱，说明测试过程和定量限结果，包括准确度和精密度验证数据。

六、线性

线性系指在设计的范围内，测定响应值结果与试样中被测物浓度直接呈比例关系的能力。

应在设计的范围内测定线性关系。可用同一对照品贮备液经精密稀释，或分别精密称取对照品，制备一系列对照品溶液的方法进行测定，至少制备 5 份不同浓度的供试样品。以测得的响应信号作为被测物浓度的函数作图，观察是否呈线性，再用最小二乘法进行线性回归。必要时，响应信号可经数学转换，再进行线性回归计算；或者可采用描述浓度 – 响应关系的非线性模型。

数据要求：应列出回归方程、相关系数和线性图（或其他数学模型）。

七、范围

范围系指分析方法能达到一定精密度、准确度和线性要求时的高低限浓度或量的区间。

范围应根据分析方法的具体应用及其线性、准确度、精密度结果和要求确定。原料药和制剂含量测定，范围一般为测定浓度的 80%～120%；制剂含量均匀度检查，范围一般为测定浓度的 70%～130%，特殊剂型，如气雾剂和喷雾剂，范围可适当放宽；溶出度或释放度中的溶出量测定，范围一般为限度的 ±30%，如规定了限度范围，则应为下限的 –20% 至上限的 +20%；杂质测定，范围应根据初步实际测定数据，拟订为规定限度的 ±20%。如果含量测定与杂质检查同时进行，用峰面积归一化法进行计算，则线性范围应为杂质规定限度的 –20% 至含量限度（或上限）的 +20%。在中药分析中，范围应根据分析方法的具体应用和线性、准确度、精密度结果及要求确定。对于有毒的、具特殊功效或药理作用的成分，其验证范围应大于被限定含量的区间。

八、耐用性

耐用性系指在测定条件有小的变动时，测定结果不受影响的承受程度，为所建立的方法用于常规检验提供依据。开始研究分析方法时，就应考虑其耐用性。如果测定试条件要求苛刻，则应在方法中写明，并注明可以接受变动的范围，可以先采用均匀设计确定主要影响因素，再通过单因素分析等确定变动范围。典型的变动因素有：被测溶液的稳定性、样品的提取次数、时间等。高效液相色谱法中典型的变动因素有：流动相的组成和 pH 值，不同品牌或不同批号的同类型色谱柱、柱温、流速等。气相色谱法变动因素有：不同品牌或批号的色谱柱、固定相、不同类型的担体、载气流速、柱温、进样口和检测器温度等。

经试验，测定条件小的变动应能满足系统适用性试验要求，以确保方法的可靠性。

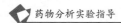

Appendix Ⅰ *Chinese Pharmacopoeia*
9101 Guidelines for Validation of Analytical Method

The purpose of validation of an analytical method is to ensure that the adopted method meets the requirements for the intended analytical applications. In the course of drafting of the drug quality specification, the analytical method must be validated. In case of changing of pharmaceutical synthetic processes or the components of preparation, or revising of the original analytical method, the analytical method of the specification must also be validated. For biological product quality control, physico-chemical analytical method and biological determination method can be employed. Because the principle of physico-chemical analytical method is applicable for both chemical and biological products, this guideline is suitable for corresponding method validation on biological product after paying special attention to their unique characteristics in the validation study. Compared to physico-chemical analytical method, more influencing factors are present in biological determination method that is out of scope of this guideline.

The analytical items that should be validated include identification, limit or quantification test, content determination (including characteristic parameters and content/potency, such as dissolution test and drug release test, etc.).

The validation indexes include specificity, accuracy, precision(including repeatability, intermediate-precision and reproducibility), detection limit, quantitation limit, linearity, range and robustness. Standard substance must be utilized in the validation of analytical method. Because of intrinsic characteristics of validation method and possible influences from analytes, the parameters to be validated should be decided depending on specific analytical method involved. The analytical items and the corresponding parameters to be validated are listed in Table 1, which can be used as a reference.

Table 1   List of validation characteristics required to be evaluated in test of each type

Parameters	Identification	Impurity test		Determination —characterisitic parameter —content of potency
		Quantitation	Limit of test	
Accuracy	–	+	–	+
Precision				

Table 1(Continued)

Parameters	Identification	Impurity test		Determination —characterisitic parameter —content of potency
		Quantitation	Limit of test	
Repeatability	–	+	–	+
Intermediate precision	–	+[①]	–	+[①]
Specificity[②]	+	+	+	+
Detection limit	–	–[③]	+	–
Quantitation limit	–	+	–	–
Linearity	–	+	–	+
Range	–	+	–	+
Robustness	+	+	+	+

① It is not necessary to validate the intermediate precision when the reproducibility has been developed.

② Lack of specificity of an individual analytical method may be compensated by other supporting analytical methods.

③ It depends on the specific condition.

The validation for the analytical method is as follow.

1　Specificity

The specificity or an analytical method is the ability to measure the analyte accurately and specifically in the presence of components that may be expected to be present in the sample matrix, such as impurities, degradation products and excipients. Specificity concerns should be investigated on identification, impurity test and content determination. If the specificity of the method is not enough, other methods with different principles should be adopted for supplementation.

1. 1　Identification

The compounds that may coexist or have close related structures should be distinguished from the active ingredient. All the samples without the tested ingredients, compounds with closely related structures and related chemical compound should produce a negative response.

1. 2　Assay and Test for Impurity

The representative graphs should be recorded for verifying specificity when chromatography or other separation methods are used. The position of each component should be marked in the graph. The resolution of the chromatographic method should meet the requirements.

If the reference substances of impurities are available, the impurities or excipients may be added to the sample for assay to inspect whether the result is interfered, and the result can be compared with that from the sample without adding impurities or excipients. As to test for impurity, a certain amount of the impurity may be added to the sample to inspect whether all ingredients including the impurity can be separated from other ingredients.

If the impurities or degradation products are not available, the sample with impurities or degradation products may be used for determination, and the result may be compared with that obtained by the pharmacopoeia method or other validated methods. Accelerating decomposition may be done for studying degradation products, such as irradiation with strong light, high temperature, high humidity, acidic or alkaline hydrolysis oxidation etc. The results of two methods should be compared for content determination and the number of impurities should be compared with that obtained in test for purity. Diode array detector and mass spectrometer may be used for purity test when necessary.

2 Accuracy

The accuracy of an analytical method is the closeness of test results obtained by that method to the true value or reference value. Accuracy is often represented as percent recovery and should be determined in the specified range.

In specified range, accuracy study should be evaluated using results form at least 6 samples of test substance at the same concentration (equivalent to 100% concentration level), or 9 samples with 3 different concentrations of testing results, the concentration range shall be considered in the setting of concentration. The purpose of analysis and the concentration range of samples should be considered in the selection of the two methods.

2.1 Accuracy of the Method for Content Determination Chemical Medicine

The accuracy for drug substance may be determined with a reference substance, or by comparing the result obtained by this method with the result obtained by another method of which the accuracy has been established. For drug preparation, its accuracy may be determined by spiking the exact amount of blank excipient in prescription dosage with known quantity of reference substance. If it is not possible to obtain all the components of excipient, the accuracy may be determined by adding known amounts of analyte to the preparation, or by comparing the result obtained by this established method with the result obtained by another method with known accuracy.

2.2 Accuracy of Quantitative Determination of Impurity for Chemical Medicine

The accuracy may be determined by spiking the drug substance or blank excipient of prescription dosage with known quantity of impurity. When the reference substance is not available for impurity or degradation product, the accuracy may be determined by comparing the result obtained by this established method with the result obtained by another matured method, such as pharmacopoeia method or validated method.

2.3 Accuracy of Determination of Ingredients for Traditional Chinese Medicine

Reference substances can be used for the determination of the recovery of added sample, e. g. certain amount of the reference substance of test substance is precisely added into the test sample with known content of analyte to be examined. The recovery ratio is calculated by margin of the determined value and the amount of the substance being examined divided by the amount of added reference substance. In the test of the recovery of added samples, the sum of the added amount of the reference substance and the amount of the analyte in the substance being examined must be in the linearity range of the standard curve. The amount of the added reference substance should be proper. A very low amount of reference substance will cause a large relative error while a high amount of reference substance will reduce the relative amount of the interference substances, so the authenticity is poor.

2. 4　Requirement for the Data

The percent recovery of the added amount, or the difference between the average value of testing results and nominal value and its relative standard deviation or confidence interval (normally at 95% confidence level) should be reported. For traditional Chinese medicine, the amount of sample used, the content of test substance in the sample, the amount of reference substance added, the testing result and calculated percent recovery, and the relative standard deviation(RSD, %) or confidence interval of percent recovery should be reported. Table 2 can be used as a reference for the relation between the content of test substance in sample and the limit of percent recovery. The limit of percent recovery can be broadened in some conditions, such as complex matrix, the content of component lower than 0. 01% and multi-components analysis.

Table 2　The content of test substance in sample and the limit of percent recovery[*]

Content of test substance in sample			Percent content in sample	Limit of percent recovery/%
%	ppm or ppb	g/mg or μg/g	g/g	
100	—	1 000 mg/g	1. 0	98 ～ 101
10	100 000 ppm	100 mg/g	0. 1	95 ～ 102
1	10 000 ppm	10 mg/g	0. 01	92 ～ 105
0. 1	1 000 ppm	1 mg/g	0. 001	90 ～ 108
0. 01	100 ppm	100 μg/g	0. 000 1	85 ～ 110
0. 001	10 ppm	10 μg/g	0. 000 01	80 ～ 115
0. 0001	1 ppm	1 μg/g	0. 000 001	75 ～ 120
—	10 ppb	0. 01 μg/g	0. 000 000 01	70 ～ 125

　＊ AOAC. *Guidelines for Single Laboratory Validation of Chemical Methods for Dietary Supplements and Botanicals.*

3 Precision

The precision of an analytical method is the closeness of agreement between a series of measurements obtained from multiple sampling of the same homogeneous sample under the prescribed conditions. The precision of an analytical method is usually expressed as deviation, standard deviation or relative standard deviation.

Repeatability is the precision obtained by the same analyst within a laboratory over a short period of time with the same equipment. Intermediate-precision is the precision obtained by different analysts within the same laboratory on different days with different equipment. Reproducibility is the precision obtained by different analysts in different laboratories using the same analytical procedure.

Precision of the method should be considered when the content of the active ingredient or impurity is determined.

3.1 Repeatability

In specified range, the repeatability of the precision study should be evaluated using results from at least 6 samples of test substance at the same concentration (equivalent to 100% concentration level), or 9 samples with 3 different concentrations of test substance and 3 test solutions at each concentration. When the repeatability is evaluated by 9 testing results, the concentration range of the sample shall be considered in the setting of the concentration.

3.2 Intermediate-Precision

A scheme should be designed to inspect the effect of random variable factors on the precision. The variable factors include different dates, different analysts and different equipments.

3.3 Reproducibility

Reproducibility should be tested when an analytical method is adopted as the national drug quality standard, for example, reproducibility should be inspected by different laboratory studies. Both the process of the collaborative study and result of the reproducibility should be recorded in the description of draft file. Where a reproducibility testing is to be conducted, the sample should be uniform, properly stored and transported to obtain reliable result.

3.4 Requirements for Data

Deviation, standard deviation, relative standard deviation and confidence interval should be reported. Table 3 can be used as a reference for the content of test substance in sample and acceptable range of the RSD for the precision (The calculation formula is $RSD_r = C^{-0.15}$ for repeatability, $RSD_R = 2C^{-0.15}$ for reproducibility, C is the content of component to be determined). Acceptable range of the RSD for the precision can be broadened in some conditions, such as complex matrix and the content of component lower than 0.01% and multi-components analysis.

Table 3   The content of test substance in sample and acceptable range of the RSD for precision*

Content of test substance in sample			Percent of content in sample	Repeatability (RSD)/%	Reproducibility (RSD)/%
%	ppm or ppb	g/mg or μg/g	g/g		
100	–	1 000 mg/g	1. 0	1	2
10	100 000 ppm	100 mg/g	0. 1	1. 5	3
1	10 000 ppm	10 mg/g	0. 01	2	4
0. 1	1 000 ppm	1 mg/g	0. 001	3	6
0. 01	100 ppm	100 μg/g	0. 000 1	4	8
0. 001	10 ppm	10 μg/g	0. 000 01	6	11
0. 0001	1 ppm	1 μg/g	0. 000 001	8	16
—	10 ppb	0. 01 μg/g	0. 000 000 01	15	32

* AOAC. *Guidelines for Single Laboratory Validation of Chemical Methods for Dietary Supplements and Botanicals.*

4   Detection Limit

Detection limit is the lowest concentration of the analyte in a sample that can be detected. The detection limit can only be used as the reference for limit test and qualitative identification, which is not applicable to quantitative analysis. The methods in common use are as follows.

4. 1   Non-instrumental Method

The detection limit is generally determined by the analysis of samples with known concentrations of analyte and by establishing the minimum level at which the analyte can be reliably detected.

4. 2   Signal-to-Noise Ratio Method

For the instrumental method recording the noise at the baseline, the lowest concentration or content of test substance that is reliably detected can be calculated by comparing the signal of sample at a known low concentration and the signal of the blank. The concentration or the amount injected into the instrument corresponding to the signal-to-noise ratio of 3 : 1 is generally accepted.

4. 3   Method of Standard Deviation and Slope of Standard Curve Based on Response Value

The detection limit is calculated by the following formula: $LOD = 3.3 \ \delta/S$. In the formula, LOD is the detection limit, δ is the standard deviation of response value, and S is the

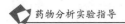

slope of standard curve. δ can be determined by following method: ①determining the standard deviation of blank; ②substituting by the residue standard deviation or the standard deviation of intercept of standard curve.

4. 4   Requirement for Data

Detection limit obtained by above methods must be validated by samples with similar content of test substance. The test graphs should be attached and the test procedures and the results of detection limit should be reported.

5   Quantitation Limit

Quantitation limit is the lowest concentration of the analyte in a sample that can be determined with acceptable precision and accuracy under the stated experimental conditions. The quantitation limit should be determined for the analytical method of micro or trace substance or the quantitative determination for impurities and degraded products. The methods in common use are as follows.

5. 1   Non-instrumental Method

Quantitation limit is generally determined by the minimum concentration or content of the analyte in a known concentration of sample that can be reliably detected.

5. 2   Signal-to-Noise Ratio Method

For the instrumental method recording the noise at the baseline, the lowest concentration or content of test substance that is reliably determined can be calculated by comparing signal of sample at a known low concentration and signal of the blank. The concentration or amount injected into the instrument corresponding to the signal-to-noise ratio of 10∶1 is generally accepted.

5. 3   Method of Standard Deviation and Slope of Standard Curve Based on Response Value

The quantitation limit is calculated by the following formula: $LOQ = 10\ \delta/S$. In the formula, LOQ is the quantitation limit, δ is the standard deviation of response value, S is the slope of standard curve. δ can be determined by following method: ①determining the standard deviation of blank; ②substituting by the residue standard deviation or the standard deviation of intercept of standard curve.

5. 4   Requirement for Data

Quantitation limit obtained by above methods must be validated by samples with similar content of test substance. The test graphs should be attached and the test procedures and the results of quantitation limit, including validation data of precision and accuracy, should be reported.

6   Linearity

The linearity of an analytical method is its ability to elicit test results that are directly proportional to the concentration of analyte in samples within a given range.

Linear relationship should be determined over the claimed range of the method. The samples with varying concentrations of analyte for linearity determination are prepared by diluting accurately a stock solution, or by measuring accurately an amount of analyte separately. At least 5 portions of samples should be prepared. The treatment is normally a calculation of a regression line by the method of least squares of test results versus analyte concentrations. In some cases, the test data may have to be subjected to mathematical transformation prior to the linearity regression analysis. It is acceptable to use a nonlinear model for concentration response relation.

Requirement for data: regression equation, correlation coefficient and the linear graph should be listed(or other mathematical models) .

7 Range

The range of an analytical method is the concentration or quantity interval between the upper and lower levels of analyte(including these levels) that have been demonstrated to be determined with precision, accuracy, and linearity using the method as written.

The range of the analytical method should be determined based on specific application of the method, its linearity accuracy and precision, and related requirement. For content determination of drug substance and preparation, the range should be 80% to 120% of the test concentration. For content uniformity of preparation, the range should be 70% to 130% of test concentration and this range may be widened appropriately for special dosage forms, such as aerosols and sprays. For dissolution test and drug release test, the range should be ±30% of the limit. If the range of limit is provided, it should be − 20% of lower limit to +20% of upper limit. For impurity determination, the range should be stipulated from −20% to +20% of the provided limit on the basis of preliminary actual determination. If the content determination and impurities test are performed simultaneously with the peak area normalization method, the linear range should be − 20 % of the provided limit of impurity to +20% of the provided limit of content(or upper limit) .

For traditional Chinese medicine, the range of analytical method should be determined based on specific application, linearity, accuracy and precision of the method, and related requirement. For toxic ingredients or those with unique efficacy or pharmacological effect, the range to be validated should be wider than the range of content.

8 Robustness

Robustness of an analytical method is the degree of tolerance that the determination result is not affected when there is small change in the operational condition. The robustness of the method should be taken into account at the beginning to develop an analytical method. If the requirement for test condition is strict, it should be recorded clearly in the method and the acceptable range of variations should be indicated. Uniform design can be used for determination of primary influencing factor then the changing range can be confirmed by single factor analysis. The typical variable factors are stability of the test solution, times and duration of sample extraction, and so on. The variable factors of liquid chromatography are composition and pH value of the mobile phase, same type of chromatographic column from different manufacturers or batches, column temperature, flow rate, etc. The variable factors of GC are column and stationary 10 hase with different brands or batches, different types of support, carrier gas flow rate, column temperature, temperature of injection port and detector, etc.

To ensure reliability of the method, the testing conditions with slight change should be confirmed to meet the requirements for system suitability.

附录二 《中国药典》《美国药典》质量标准选读（以对乙酰氨基酚原料为例）
Appendix Ⅱ Selecting Monograph from ChP and USP（Take Paracetamol as an Example）

《中国药典》（2020 年版）二部，第 386 页。

对乙酰氨基酚（《中国药典》）

Duiyixian'anjifen

Paracetamol

$C_8H_9NO_2$ 151.16

本品为 4'-羟基乙酰苯胺。按干燥品计算，含 $C_8H_9NO_2$ 应为 98.0%～102.0%。

【性状】 本品为白色结晶或结晶性粉末；无臭。

本品在热水或乙醇中易溶，在丙酮中溶解，在水中略溶。

熔点 本品的熔点（通则 0612）为 168 ～ 172 ℃。

【鉴别】 （1）本品的水溶液加三氯化铁试液，即显蓝紫色。

（2）取本品约 0.1 g，加稀盐酸 5 mL，置水浴中加热 40 min，放冷；取 0.5 mL，滴加亚硝酸钠试液 5 滴，摇匀，用水 3 mL 稀释后，加碱性 β-萘酚试液 2 mL，振摇，即显红色。

（3）本品的红外光谱应与对照的图谱（光谱集 131 图）一致。

【检查】 **酸度** 取本品 0.10 g，加水 10 mL 使溶解，依法测定（通则 0631），pH 应为 5.5 ～ 6.5。

乙醇溶液的澄清度与颜色 取本品 1.0 g，加乙醇 10 mL 溶解后，溶液应澄清，无色；如显浑浊，与 1 号浊度标准液（通则 0902 第一法）比较，不得更浓；如显色，与棕红色 2 号或橙红色 2 号标准比色液（通则 0901 第一法）比较，不得更深。

氯化物 取本品 2.0 g，加水 100 mL，加热溶解后，冷却，滤过，取滤液 25 mL，依法检查（通则 0801），与标准氯化钠溶液 5.0 mL 制成的对照液比较，不得更浓（0.01%）。

硫酸盐　取氯化物项下剩余的滤液 25 mL，依法检查（通则 0802），与标准硫酸钾溶液 1.0 mL 制成的对照液比较，不得更浓（0.02%）。

有关物质　照高效液相色谱法（通则 0512）测定。临用新制。

溶剂　甲醇－水（4∶6）。

供试品溶液　取本品适量，精密称定，加溶剂溶解并定量稀释制成每毫升中约含 20 mg 的溶液。

对照品溶液　取对氨基酚对照品适量，精密称定，加溶剂溶解并定量稀释制成每 1 mL 中约含 0.1mg 的溶液。

对照溶液　精密量取对照品溶液与供试品溶液各 1 mL，置同一 100 mL 量瓶中，用溶剂稀释至刻度，摇匀。

色谱条件　用辛基硅烷键合硅胶为填充剂；以磷酸盐缓冲液（取磷酸氢二钠8.95 g，磷酸二氢钠3.9 g，加水溶解至 1 000 mL，加 10 % 四丁基氢氧化铵溶液 12 mL）—甲醇（90∶10）为流动相；检测波长为 245 nm；柱温为 40 ℃；进样体积为 20 μL。

系统适用性要求　理论板数按对乙酰氨基酚峰计算不低于 2 000。对氨基酚峰与对乙酰氨基酚峰之间的分离度应符合要求。

测定法　精密量取供试品溶液与对照溶液，分别注入液相色谱仪，记录色谱图至主峰保留时间的 4 倍。

限度　供试品溶液色谱图中如有与对氨基酚保留时间一致的色谱峰，按外标法以峰面积计算，含对氨基酚不得超过 0.005%，其他单个杂质峰面积不得大于对照溶液中对乙酰氨基酚峰面积的 0.1 倍（0.1%），其他各杂质峰面积的和不得大于对照溶液中对乙酰氨基酚峰面积的 0.5 倍（0.5%）。

对氯苯乙酰胺　照高效液相色谱法（通则 0512）测定。临用新制。

溶剂与供试品溶液　见有关物质项下。

对照品溶液　取对氯苯乙酰胺对照品与对乙酰氨基酚对照品各适量，精密称定，加溶剂溶解并定量稀释制成每毫升中约含对氯苯乙酰胺 1 μg 与对乙酰氨基酚 20 μg 的混合溶液。

色谱条件　用辛基硅烷键合硅胶为填充剂；以磷酸盐缓冲液（取磷酸氢二钠 8.95 g，磷酸二氢钠3.9 g，加水溶解至 1 000 mL，加 10% 四丁基氢氧化按 12 mL）－甲醇（60∶40）为流动相；检测波长为 245 nm；柱温为 40 ℃；进样体积为 20 μL。

系统适用性要求　理论板数按对乙酰氨基酚峰计算不低于 2 000。对氯苯乙酰胺峰与对乙酰氨基酚峰之间的分离度应符合要求。

测定法　精密量取供试品溶液与对照品溶液，分别注入液相色谱仪，记录色谱图。

限度　按外标法以峰面积计算，含对氯苯乙酰胺不得超过 0.005%。

干燥失重　取本品，在 105 ℃ 干燥至恒重，减失重量不得超过 0.5%（通则 0831）。

炽灼残渣　不得超过 0.1%（通则 0841）。

重金属 取本品 1.0 g，加水 20 mL，置水浴中加热使溶解放冷，滤过，取滤液加醋酸盐缓冲液（pH 3.5）2 mL 与水适量使成 25 mL，依法检查（通则 0821 第一法），含重金属不得过百万分之十。

【含量测定】 取本品约 40 mg，精密称定，置 250 mL 量瓶中，加 0.4% 氢氧化钠溶液 50 mL 溶解后，加水至刻度，摇匀，精密量取 5 mL，置 100 mL 量瓶中，加 0.4% 氢氧化钠溶液 10 mL，加水至刻度，摇匀。

测定法 取供试品溶液，在 257 nm 的波长处测定吸收度，按 $C_8H_9NO_2$ 的吸收系数（$E_{cm}^{1\%}$）为 715 计算，即得。

【类别】 解热镇痛、非甾体抗炎药。

【贮藏】 密封保存。

【制剂】 ①对乙酰氨基酚片；②对乙酰氨基酚咀嚼片；③对乙酰氨基酚泡腾片；④对乙酰氨基酚注射液；⑤对乙酰氨基酚栓；⑥对乙酰氨基酚胶囊；⑦对乙酰氨基酚颗粒；⑧对乙酰氨基酚滴剂；⑨对乙酰氨基酚凝胶。

USP-NF, 2019

Acetaminophen(USP)

$C_8H_9NO_2$ 151.16

Acetamide, N-(4-hydroxyphenyl) -4'-Hydroxyacetanilide [103 – 90 – 2].

Acetaminophen contains not less than 98.0 percent and not more than 101.0 percent of $C_8H_9NO_2$, calculated on the anhydrous basis.

Packaging and storage — Preserve in tight, light-resistant containers, and store at room temperature. Protect from moisture and heat.

USP Reference standards‹11›

USP Acetaminophen RS.

Identification—

A: Infrared Absorption ‹197K›.

B: Ultraviolet Absorption ‹197U›.

Solution: 5 μg/mL.

Medium: 0.1 N hydrochloric acid in methanol(1 in 100).

C: It responds to the *Thin-layer Chromatographic Identification Test* ‹201›, a test solution in methanol containing about 1 mg/mL and a solvent system consisting of a mixture of methylene chloride and methanol(4 : 1) being used.

Melting range ⟨**741**⟩ between 168 and 172.

Water, Method I ⟨**921**⟩ not more than 0. 5%.

Residue on ignition ⟨**281**⟩ not more than 0. 1%.

Chloride‹221›— Shake 1. 0 g with 25 mL of water, filter, and add 1 mL of 2 N nitric acid and 1 mL of silver nitrate TS: the filtrate shows no more chloride than corresponds to 0. 20 mL of 0. 020 N hydrochloric acid(0. 014%).

Sulfate ⟨**221**⟩ — Shake 1. 0 g with 25 mL of water, filter, add 2 mL of 1 N acetic acid, then add 2 mL of barium chloride TS: the mixture shows no more sulfate than corresponds to 0. 20 mL of 0. 020 N sulfuric acid(0. 02%).

Sulfide— Place about 2. 5 g in a 50 mL beaker. Add 5 mL of alcohol and 1 mL of 3 N hydrochloric acid. Moisten a piece of lead acetate test paper with water, and fix to the underside of a watch glass. Cover the beaker with the watch glass so that part of the lead acetate paper hangs down near the pouring spout of the beaker. Heat the contents of the beaker on a hot plate just to boiling: no coloration or spotting of the test paper occurs.

Heavy metals, Method Ⅱ ‹231› 0. 001%.

Free *p*-aminophenol— Transfer 5. 0 g to a 100 mL volumetric flask, and dissolve in about 75 mL of a mixture of equal volumes of methanol and water. Add 5. 0 mL of alkaline nitroferricyanide solution(prepared by dissolving 1 g of sodium nitroferricyanide and 1 g of anhydrous sodium carbonate in 100 mL of water), dilute with a mixture of equal volumes of methanol and water to volume, mix, and allow to stand for 30 min. Concomitantly determine the absorbances of this solution and of a freshly prepared solution of *p*-aminophenol, similarly prepared at a concentration of 25 μg/mL, using the same quantities of the same reagents, in 1 cm cells, at the maximum at about 710 nm, with a suitable spectrophotometer, using 5. 0 mL of alkaline nitroferricyanide solution diluted with a mixture of equal volumes of methanol and water to 100 mL as the blank: The absorbance of the test solution does not exceed that of the standard solution, corresponding to not more than 0. 005% of p-aminophenol.

Limit of p-chloroacetanilide— Transfer 1. 0 g to a glass-stoppered, 15 mL centrifuge tube, add 5. 0 mL of ether, shake by mechanical means for 30 minutes, and centrifuge at 1 000 rpm for 15 minutes or until a clean separation is obtained. Apply 200 μL of the supernatant, in 40 μL portions, to obtain a single spot not more than 10 mm in diameter to a suitable thin-layer chromatographic plate(see Chromatography ‹621›) coated with a 0. 25 mm layer of chromatographic silica gel mixture. Similarly apply 40 μL of a standard solution in ether containing 10 μg of p-chloroacetanilide per mL, and allow the spots to dry. Develop the chromatogram in an unsaturated chamber, with a solvent system consisting of a mixture of solvent hexane and acetone(75 : 25), until the solvent front has moved three-fourths of the length of the plate. Remove the plate from the developing chamber, mark the solvent front, and allow the solvent to evaporate. Locate the spots in the chromatogram by examination under short-wavelength UV light: Any spot obtained from the solution under test, at an *RF* value corresponding to the principal spot from the standard solution, is not greater in size or intensity than the principal spot obtained from the standard solution, corresponding to not more than 0.001% of p-chloroacetanilide.

Readily carbonizable substances‹271› — Dissolve 0.50 g in 5 mL of sulfuric acid TS: the solution has no more color than Matching Fluid A.

Assay— Dissolve about 120 mg of acetaminophen, accurately weighed, in 10 mL of methanol in a 500 mL volumetric flask, dilute with water to volume, and mix. Transfer 5.0 mL of this solution to a 100 mL volumetric flask, dilute with water to volume, and mix. Concomitantly determine the absorbances of this solution and of a standard solution of USP Acetaminophen RS, in the same medium, at a concentration of about 12 μg/mL in 1 cm cells, at the wavelength of maximum absorbance at about 244 nm, with a suitable spectrophotometer, using water as the blank. Calculate the quantity, in mg, of $C_8H_9NO_2$ in the acetaminophen taken by the formula:

$$10C\ (A_U/A_S)$$

in which C is the concentration, in μg per mL, of USP Acetaminophen RS in the standard solution; and A_U and A_S are the absorbances of the solution of Acetaminophen and the standard solution, respectively.

附录三　药物分析常用英语词汇
Appendix Ⅲ　Vocabulary Commonly Used in Pharmaceutical Analysis

容器类（vessel）

比色皿 cuvette
比重瓶 specific gravity bottle
表面皿 watch glass
不锈钢杯 stainless-steel beaker
称量瓶 weighing bottle
碘量瓶 iodine flask
分液漏斗 separating funnel
坩埚 crucible
广口瓶 wide-mouth bottle
刻度移液管 graduated pipettes
冷凝管 condenser
量杯 measuring cup
量筒 measuring flask/cylinder
漏斗 funnel
滤管 filter
锥形瓶 conical flask
培养皿 culture dish
容量瓶 volumetric flask/measuring flask
烧杯 beaker
烧瓶 flask
试管 test tube
试剂瓶 reagent bottles
吸液管 pipette
洗耳球 rubber suction bulb
洗瓶 plastic wash bottle
小滴管 dropper
蒸发皿 evaporating dish
蒸馏烧瓶 distilling flask

实验用器材（equipment）

白大褂 white gown
玻棒 glass rod
玻璃活塞 stopcock
擦镜纸 wiper for lens
称量纸 weighing paper
磁力搅拌器 magnetic stirrer
打孔器 stopper borer
滴定管 burette
电动搅拌器 electronic blender
电极 electrode
电炉 heater
电炉丝 wire coil for heater
电热套 heating mantle
电泳槽 electrophoresis tank
沸石 boiling stone
复印纸 copy paper
盖玻片 cover glass
坩埚钳 crucible tong/crucible clamp
活塞 piston
记号笔 marker pen
剪刀 scissor
碱式滴定管 burette for alkali
搅拌棒 stirring rod
搅拌装置 stirring device
酒精灯 alcohol burner
酒精喷灯 blast alcohol burner
口罩 respirator
垃圾袋 disposable bag
离心管 centrifuge tube

铝箔 aluminium foil
玛瑙研钵 agate mortar
闹钟 alarm clock
黏度计 viscometer
镊子 forceps/tweezers
塞子 stopper
筛子 sieve
试管架 test tube holder/rack
试管刷 test-tube brush
手术刀 scalpel
水银温度计 mercury thermometer
脱脂棉 absorbent cotton
万能夹 extension clamp
橡胶管 rubber tubing
橡皮筋 rubber band
研杵 pestle
阳极/正极 anode
药匙 lab spoon
移液枪 pipette
移液枪枪头 pipette tips
阴极/负极 cathode
游码 crossbeams and sliding weights
圆形漏斗架 cast-iron ring
载玻片 slide
注射器 syringe

仪器（instrument）

CO_2 培养箱 CO_2 incubator
PCR 仪 PCR amplifier
X 射线衍射仪 X-ray diffractometer
超临界流体色谱仪 supercritical fluid chromatograph
超低温冰箱 ultra-low temperature freezer
电子俘获检测器 electron capture detector, ECD
分析天平 analytical balance
傅里叶变换红外光谱仪 Fourier transform infrared spectrometer, FTIR spectrometer

高效液相色谱仪 high performance (pressure) liquid chromatograph, HPLC
光学显微镜 optical microscopy
核磁共振波谱仪 nuclear magnetic resonance spectrometer/NMR
恒温循环泵 constant temperature circulator
离心机 centrifuge
粒度分析仪 particle size analyzer
凝胶渗透色谱仪 gel permeation chromatograph
气相色谱仪 gas chromatograph
气相色谱 – 质谱联用仪 gas chromatograph-mass spectrometer, GC-MS
热分析仪 thermal analyzer
熔点测定仪 melting point tester
酸式滴定管 acid burette
天平 balance/scale
旋光仪 polarimeter
液相色谱 – 质谱联用仪 liquid chromato-graphy-mass spectrometry, LC-MS
原子发射光谱仪 atomic emission spectrometer
原子吸收光谱仪 atomic absorption spectrometer
折光计 refractometer
真空泵 vacuum pump
紫外检测仪 ultraviolet detector
紫外可见分光光度计 UV-visible spectrophotometer

分析数据处理（data processing of analysis）

变异系数 coefficient of variation
标准偏差（标准差）standard deviation, SD
定量限 limit of quantitation, LOQ
范围 range

回收率 recovery

检测限 limit of detection，LOD

检查 test

精密度 precision

空白试验 blank test

灵敏度 sensitivity

耐用性 robustness

随机误差 accidental error

误差 absolute error

系统误差 systematic error

线性 linearity

相对平均偏差 relative standard deviation，RSD

相对误差 relative error

校正因子 correction factor

信噪比 signal-to-noise ratio

有效数字 significant figure

置信水平 confidence level

中间精密度 intermediate-precision

重复性 repeatability

重现性 reproducibility

专属性 specificity

准确度 accuracy

实验操作（manipulation）

超声破碎 ultrasonication

沉淀 precipitate

淬灭 quench

点样 apply

电泳 electrophoresis

丢弃 discard

分解 decomposition/dissolution

分装 aliquot

孵育 incubate

过滤 filtrate

蒸馏 distil/distill

搅拌 stir/agitate

接种 inoculate

均质化 homogenize

冷却 chill down

离心收集 pellet

灭菌 sterilize

浓缩 condense

培养 foster

漂洗 rinse

平衡 equilibrate

鉴别 identification

破碎 crush

切碎 chop/mince

溶解 dissolve

上样 load the sample

通风 ventilate

脱水 dehydrate

涡旋震荡 vortex

吸出 aspirate

稀释 dilute

洗脱 elute

校准 calibrate

絮状沉淀 flocculent precipitate

旋转 swirl/ spin

研磨 grind

氧化 oxidize

展开 develop

实验方法（method）

薄层色谱法 thin layer chromatography，TLC

差式扫描量热法 differential scanning calorimetry，DSC

超临界流体萃取 supercritical fluid extraction，SFE

超临界流体色谱法 supercritical fluid chromatography

碘量法 iodometric titration

电感耦合等离子发射光谱法 inductively

coupled plasma atomic
emission spectrometry
电泳法 electrophoresis
费休氏水分测定法 Karl Fischer titration
过程反应分析 in-process reaction analysis
过程分析 process analytical technology
红外吸收光谱法 infrared spectroscopy，IR
化学计量学 chemometrics
拉曼光谱法 roman spectrometry
离子色谱法 ion chromatography
联用技术 combination techniques

络合滴定法 complexometric titration
毛细管电泳法 capillary electrophoresis
体积排阻色谱法 size exclusion
chromatography
氧化还原滴定 redox titration
荧光分光光度法 fluorescence
spectrophotometry
质谱法 mass spectrometry
紫外可见分光光度法 ultraviolet-visible
spectrophoto-metry

参 考 文 献

［1］国家药典委员会. 中华人民共和国药典（2020 年版）［M］. 北京：中国医药科技出版社，2020.

［2］杭太俊. 药物分析［M］. 8 版. 北京：人民卫生出版社，2016.

［3］中国食品药品检定研究院. 中国药品检验标准操作规范（2019 年版）［M］. 北京：中国医药科技出版社，2019.

［4］中国药品生物制品检定所. 药品检验仪器操作规程（2010 年）［M］. 北京：中国医药科技出版社，2010.

［5］British Pharmacopoeia Commission. British pharmacopoeia（2020）［M］. 2020.

［6］The United States pharmacopeial convention USP – NF 2019 ［M］. 2019.

［7］The European directorate for the quality of medicines. EP 10. 0 ［M］. 2020.